How to get a job in medicine

Adam Poole BSc MBBS MRCS

Director, Arcus
London, UK

Chapter 12 contributed by

Manoj Ramachandran BSc MBBS MRCS

Specialist Registrar in Trauma and Orthopaedics
Royal National Orthopaedic Hospital Middlesex, UK

Illustrations by
David Banks

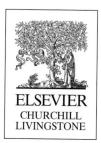

ELSEVIER
CHURCHILL
LIVINGSTONE

EDINBURGH LONDON NEW YORK OXFORD PHILADELPHIA ST LOUIS SYDNEY TORONTO 2005

ELSEVIER
CHURCHILL
LIVINGSTONE

© 2005, Adam Poole.

First published 2005

ISBN 0-443-10014-4

British Library Cataloguing in Publication Data
A catalogue record for this book is available from the British Library

Library of Congress Cataloging in Publication Data
A catalog record for this book is available from the Library of Congress

Working together to grow
libraries in developing countries

www.elsevier.com | www.bookaid.org | www.sabre.org

ELSEVIER   BOOK AID International   Sabre Foundation

your source for books,
journals and multimedia
in the health sciences
www.elsevierhealth.com

The
publisher's
policy is to use
**paper manufactured
from sustainable forests**

Printed in China

Preface

It's easy to underperform by being unprepared. Jobs in medicine are increasingly competitive, driven by a 60% increase in the number of graduates in the UK, more overseas-trained doctors taking up posts here, and higher expectations from both employers and patients. Whether applying for an SHO or Foundation post, many doctors make numerous job applications without success. For some, the stumbling block is being shortlisted in the first place. In other cases a potentially winning CV is stymied by poor interview technique.

Like many aspects of a medical career, the old fashioned view is that CVs and interviews are things you should be able to just 'do'. Training, such as would be expected for clinical or technical development, has been considered unnecessary by the medical establishment and possibly the wider NHS. This view is changing rapidly because the NHS has accepted the evidence from the corporate world that developing individuals to their maximum potential makes them better at their jobs. Whether in management, leadership or career development, it can be proved that success can be nurtured and isn't just innate.

But, equally, there is a complacent view among some candidates that the 'best' person will always get the job. This assumption has no solid basis in fact. There is no doubt that the 'favourite' for the job is frequently pipped to the post by another challenger who is better prepared.

This book shows you how to make the leap from a random approach to the job application process, to creating a successful CV and interviewing really well. It is intended to be suitable for everyone. Some readers who are very experienced at applications might find parts of the content obvious but hopefully there will be many points you will not have previously considered. The book is designed to open your mind, to challenge assumptions and to consider what objectives you should set and how to meet them. It is not an encyclopaedia of lists of questions but rather a practical guide that will benefit you quickly, economically and as efficiently as possible.

The application process is clearly broken down into four sections: CV writing, compiling application forms, interview technique and the specialist types of job selection.

Recruiters spend eight seconds looking at medical CVs. That isn't long to impress. Many people erroneously think that the CV is simply a long list: a kind of index of an individual's past. In fact, the CV is used to sell you to the recruiter. This book explores specific successful ways to change a boring CV into an inspiring sales aid.

As application forms have been added to the selection process I explain why they are dangerous traps that need to be treated with great caution. Deft hints on how to get past awkward questions are discussed. A unique and definitive research project has looked at hundreds of medical application forms, identifying for the first time the most common questions asked.

There is nothing better than leaving an interview feeling that you have done a great job. The book defines which parts of an interview can – and should – be prepared for; suggests how to manage nerves and explains what to do if the interview seems to be going badly.

Being prepared includes a familiarity with the format of the interview. Success doesn't come from answering questions as if grabbing apples from the nearest low-hanging branch. Instead, understanding why certain questions are asked dictates how they are best answered. It isn't possible to list all the questions that you might ever be asked and personally I wouldn't believe or buy a book that made that claim. But what I have done is to categorise the possibilities and demonstrate ways of dealing with all the potential styles of questioning.

The ideal outcome from reading this book is that you feel more confident and prepared. A brilliant outcome would be that – more confident and better prepared – you actually enjoy the job application process. After all, you are going to have to undergo job selection many, many times during a long career. Why not enjoy it?

Thank you for buying and reading the book. If you have any comments on it please e-mail them to me at adam.poole@arcus.co.uk.

AP

Acknowledgements

The initial inspiration for my fascination with great CVs and interview technique came from an early mentor who has not been involved in the completion of this book at all. Dr Annette Steele was instrumental in making me think differently about the importance of the CV as a sales tool and in believing that interview technique could both be taught and improved.

I would like to thank Dr Paul Dilworth for diligently and patiently working on many CV and interview training courses with me. Dr Bob Edenborough from the management consulting firm KPMG has written a fascinating study of the process of interviewing (*Effective Interviewing*) and has spent a great deal of time discussing the intricacies of exceptional interviewing and selection with me. My two great researchers, James Blackburn and Steve Kahane, worked very hard in collecting and analysing application forms for the content of Chapter 6. My colleague Mr Andrew Tasker was constructive in working through the language used to ensure it was appropriate.

Dr Radegund Norbury helped enormously with the chapter on GP career progression. Psychologist Dr Caroline Elton gave me a balanced and informed view of non-interview selection and of career progression in general. Dr Rhona MacDonald and Dr Graham Easton from the BMJ have fostered a great deal of debate on selection and interviewing, including commissioning a number of articles that have provoked interest and analysis. At GlaxoSmithKline (GST) my previous colleagues Phil Russell and Dr Helen Price motivated me to think about the importance of organisational and team development and culture.

I would also thank my mother, Anne, for help with the English grammar and syntax and, finally, Laurence Hunter and Hannah Kenner at Elsevier. Laurence believed in the project and worked really hard through a great deal of planning to make it happen; Hannah kept me on track and on time in the project's delivery.

Contents

1 CVs and application forms 1
A two-stage process 2
Researching this book 4

2 Starting the CV with a blank sheet 6
It's all sales 7
Getting started 8
No 'right way' 9
The blank sheet 9
What are the buyers in the market to buy? 10
Past performance predicts future performance 11
An example of 'success' 11
Adding flesh to your achievements:
    Positive Power Verbs 12

3 The front page 15
Title: branding the rest of the paper 17
Headlines 18
Which direction? 19
It's what you did 19
Dates 21
Trailers 21
Big hitters 21
What can't you read? 23

4 Employment and education 25
What goes first? 25
Fixed and variable achievements 26
Employment 28
Advanced selling 30
Linking jobs together 30
Education 30
How to sell educational qualifications 31

5 **Adding depth to the CV: the second page** 33
Transferable skills 34
Management and leadership 34
Academic background 35
Academic publications 36
Presentations 37
Prizes and awards 38
Clinical governance 38
Patient focused 40
Teamworking, relationship building and
   multiprofessional work 40
The end of the CV: interests and references 41

6 **Researching application forms** 44
Scope of research 44
Obtaining the forms: written advertisements and
   internet versions 45
Time to closing date 47
Application by CV 47
Typical application forms 49
What are the different subsections of application
   forms? 49

7 **Introduction to application forms and the
link to the CV** 54
Negative experience 55
Over applying 55
Opening the application form 56

8 **Filling in the application form** 58
Saving time 58
Principles of selling using application forms 59
Multiple applications 60
Introducing big hitters 61
Being positive: what are the benefits of the
   application form to the job seeker? 61
Your own handwriting 63
Extra pages 63

9 Top 20 application form questions 64
Academic background 64
Clinical experience and achievements 66
Teaching 69
Management 70
Personal criteria 71

10 Summary of CVs and application forms 75
Review 75
When is it finished? 75
Final checks 77
Getting opinions 77
Before putting the application into the post 78
Covering letter 78
Increasing your chances after your application
has been received 79
How to make your pack look the best 79
Contacting the recruiter 81

11 The interview 82
Stages of execution of the winning interview 83
Making time 84
Interview questions 84
Common myths about interviews – all are false 85

12 Preparation for the interview 87
by Manoj Ramachandran
Preparing for the interview once shortlisted 88
The interview format 89
The interview panel 89
What are your odds? 90
Practise, practise, practise 90
Preparing on the day of the interview 91
You are you being watched . . . 92
Don't forget . . . 93
What you see is what you get (WYSIWYG) 94

13 How do they decide?   97
How do you get a job?   97
What is the panel looking for?   98
What if they have already made up their minds?   99
How can you tell if the panel isn't really giving you
   a look-in?   100
Internal candidates   101
Interview selection theory   102
Selection panels   104

14 5 minutes before and 1 minute after   107
Stress building up   107
5 minutes to go   107
Delays and hold-ups   108
Walking through the door   110
Shaking hands   110
Sitting down   110
The last minute of the interview   111

15 Open/retrospective questions   114
Open/retrospective questions   114
Basic principles   115
Recognising the style   116
Common pitfalls   116
Common questions   118
Polishing your technique   120

16 Topical questions   124
Basic principles   125
Recognising the style   126
Common pitfalls   127
Common questions   128
Polishing technique   129

17 Aggressive/closed questions   133
Basic principles   134
Recognising the style   136
Common pitfalls   137

Common questions		138
Polishing technique		140

18 Specific types of medical job application 143
Academic jobs 143
The CV and application form 144
Paper qualifications 144
Publications 145
Presentations 145
The interview 146
Interviews with 'bolt-ons' 146

19 Closing the interview and following up 151
Anything to ask us? 151
Finishing the interview 153
Good news: you've been successful 154
Bad news: you have not been successful 155

20 Summary of interviews 158
Combination interviews 158
Moving from style to style 159
Most common pitfalls to avoid in all styles of
interview 160
Honing your personal technique: ten last tips 162

21 General practice 164
What's different? 164
Switching into general practice training 165
GP registrar year 166
Substantive GP posts 166
Topical interview questions 167

22 Assessment tools 169
Why are assessment tools used? 169
What kinds of assessment tools are there? 170
Personality testing (psychometrics) 171
360-degree evaluation 172
In-tray exercises 173
Preparing for assessment exercises 173

23 The future of medical selection   175
   Drivers for change   176
   Predictions for the future   177

Appendix 1 **Medical grades**   180
Foundation programme grade   181
Non-standard grade (Trust) doctors   181

Appendix 2 **Where do you go to find a job?**   183
UK Deaneries   183

Appendix 3 **Further reading**   185
Selected bibliography   185

Index   187

CVs and application forms

In this chapter

- What is the process for gaining a medical job in the UK?
- How are CVs and application forms used in practice?
- How have we gone about researching for this book to analyse current practice and identify trends?

Career progression in medicine is different from in any other walk of life. At every stage prior to the award of a substantive consultant or GP post, jobs have time limits. The system of training in the UK requires doctors to reapply for posts as frequently as every six months. There are no exceptions and the following pattern is typical for the average hospital doctor:

Pre-registration	One rotation or two jobs
Foundation programmes	Likely to be one rotation (from August 2005)
SHO posts	One rotation or four to five jobs
Post-membership posts	Two to four jobs
Research posts	One job
Pre-SpR posts	One to three jobs
SpR jobs	One rotation
Consultant posts	One job

Just to get through medical training you need to be successful in at least eight selection processes. This does not include applications that are unsuccessful, and I have not met a single consultant who had a clean sweep and got every single job he or she applied for.

So medical graduates need to become uniquely expert at presenting their CVs and interviewing for jobs. But most Trusts never coach their medical staff in either of these areas.

Myths abound about the 'correct' way of completing a CV, and the 'right' way to interview for jobs. In developing and researching this book, I sought the truth. The truth is always surprising to some: and some of the findings described certainly surprised me. But it's only in handling the truth that you will become really successful in marketing yourself and getting the jobs you want.

There is also a huge amount of negativity in the jobseekers' world. Some doctors repeatedly fail to be shortlisted. Others get to the interview and don't succeed. Many have been told not to bother applying because they won't be successful. And those coming into the UK system from other countries describe episodes of bemusement at the requirements of NHS Trusts, and sometimes even a degree of prejudice.

A TWO-STAGE PROCESS

The first truth is that the medical job application process is always in two stages:

CV/application form → Shortlisted for interview → Job offer

There is no way of bypassing either of these stages and, for the purposes of dividing the book up, they are considered entirely separately.

CVs and application forms

CVs are used much more frequently than application forms throughout the medical career. As well as being used for the job selection process they are needed for:

- annual appraisal
- record of in-service training assessments (RITA)
- career portfolios
- deanery monitoring of training.

The application form, on the other hand, is entirely specific for the job selection process. Approximately three-quarters of medical jobs require the completion of an application form: the rest are application by CV only.

CVs are better for the candidate and application forms are better for the employing Trusts. This is because the design of the CV is up to you. It is your decision where to put things, what to emphasise, what to describe and what simply to list, and how to use your previous history to your advantage. In some ways it is similar to being the producer on the 10 o'clock news. You can order the segments in exactly the way you want to – to emphasise certain stories that you want to bring out.

Ask the expert

I have been told there is a standard format for completing a CV – could you provide me with that format?

No, because there isn't one. The job application process is an art and not a science. Unlike the requirements of the job itself – where you follow guidelines, medical evidence and clinical knowledge – there is no specific format. In other words, you decide how to set out your own CV. Don't be tempted to simply take someone else's CV and reproduce it. You won't be successful.

The requirements for completing a CV – for any of its uses – are different from application forms and are considered in Chapters 2, 3, 4 and 5. Application forms are examined in Chapters 6, 7, 8 and 9.

Ask the expert
How long?
As this is one of the questions I'm asked most, I'm putting my view on the most appropriate length of the CV here in Chapter 1.
Everybody worries about the length of their CV. The CVs I have seen vary enormously. I once saw a CV for a year 1 SHO post that was 24 pages long. One of the most common reasons for a CV being overlong is that it tends to have huge amounts of space on every page, and lots of subheadings. Neither are necessary - as I will demonstrate in the coming chapters.

Top Tip
The CV should be *as short as possible*. Two opposing factors influence length of the CV:
1. It should not contain any irrelevant ancient history or extraneous information: editing these things will shorten the CV.
2. It must sell your achievements and so cannot simply be a list of what you have done: this tends to lengthen the CV.

Most CVs can easily be successful at two sides long; at most four. However, listing a number of academic publications is one of the more common (and better) reasons for a long CV. Really good ways of handling this are dealt with later.

RESEARCHING THIS BOOK

Although much of this book is informed by experience of medical CVs and interviews, one section required particular analysis. Application forms are not something people normally ask me to review, and I have rarely been involved with their creation. So a research team gathered 200 job application packs and analysed every single application form. I'm not aware this has ever been done before and the results of this exhaustive and inevitably time-consuming research are detailed in Chapter 6.

Summary

- The best that can be achieved by an awesome application form and a champion CV is to be shortlisted for interview

- Plan for a CV that is 2 sides long

- Never try to use someone else's format to produce your own CV

Starting the CV with a blank sheet

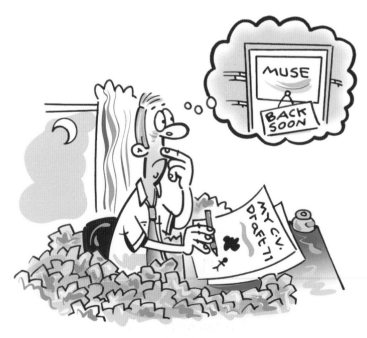

2

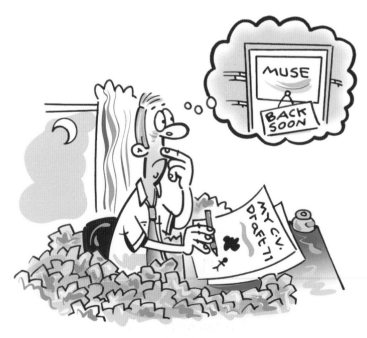

In this chapter

- How do you start writing your CV?

- How do you modify an existing CV to make it relevant for the purpose for which it is now required?

- Why you need to sell yourself – and how do you do it with a CV?

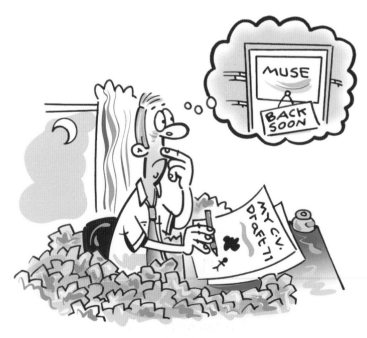

'Where do I start?'

The two-stage model for success in medical job applications is:

CV/application form → Shortlisted for interview → Job offer

The objective of a CV is to get shortlisted. It's important to bear this in mind because very often you are tempted to put too much information onto the CV, which reduces its impact. If employers want more information about something you have done in the past they can ask for the detail at the interview.

IT'S ALL SALES

To succeed in obtaining competitive jobs, applicants need to sell themselves to recruiters. The jobseeker is the seller and the employer the buyer. The more competitive the job, the greater the need for the applicant to sell to the buyer.

Doctors don't like to sell themselves. It's seen as grubby, not part of the culture: medicine isn't a sales job. But in selling yourself, you will get noticed by the readers of the CV and shortlisted. And don't forget once again that the CV has only one objective – to get you shortlisted.

What are you selling?

You need to consider what the buyers are in the market to buy. It isn't as simple as saying 'an SHO' or 'an SpR' because if they wanted just any available SpR they would simply draw lots among all the candidates and randomly allocate the job. Employers always have the choice between candidates and can use whatever criteria they like to select from the pool.

Successful candidates predict what the buyers are looking for and ensure that their CV demonstrates that they have the relevant portfolio of skills and achievements to get shortlisted.

You are selling *achievements*: it would be very odd to sell failures. You are not trying to generate a boring list of what you have done but instead a stimulating insight into your past that leaves the readers *wanting more information*. They get this information at the interview.

The whole of the CV needs to sell your achievements to the buyers but the most important part of all is the front page of the CV.

Why? Because buyers are very impatient.

Impatient buyers

 Top Tip
The average medical CV is read in 8 seconds.

Reviewers of CVs have a huge number to look through. They take an average of 8 seconds to read a CV. You have 8 seconds to impress someone enough to place your CV into the 'shortlist' pile rather than the 'reject' pile. It follows that the more applicants for the post, the more quickly the CV will be read.

If buyers have to search for information it is much easier for them simply to reject you. It's too much hassle for them to find detail they need if it's hidden away. Your first task in selling yourself efficiently is to *anticipate* what the impatient buyer will require and present that information in a straightforward way.

GETTING STARTED

Ask yourself the question: 'What do I really want the recruiter to know about me?' Although friends and current colleagues can make suggestions, it's you who must decide what is put in and what is left out.

NO 'RIGHT WAY'

People often ask about the right way to present a CV. What order things should be in, what font and what type size. The truth is there isn't a correct way to do any of these things. It is definitely an art rather than a science. Ultimately, it is your decision how you want to lay out the information.

Convention dictates certain things to help you. For instance that dates are always placed in *reverse chronological order* – starting with the most recent event and working backwards. The buyer is much more interested in your MD than your GCSE results.

But other aspects of a 'conventional' CV are hopelessly out-dated. The worst CVs have a first page containing an elongated list of contact details surrounded by loads of empty space. You have no chance of selling yourself with your phone number and e-mail address and are wasting valuable time by making the buyer turn over page after page after page to find something interesting to read about you.

 Don't put a covering page over your CV with the words 'curriculum vitae' on it. Everyone knows it's a CV and it's the first page that sells you most efficiently, so use it to its greatest possible effect.

THE BLANK SHEET

First, whenever you have to write a CV, begin with a blank sheet of paper. Don't just dust down the CV you submitted 5 years ago and add a few changes. You will think differently now about which successes over your career you want to sell. And the objective of this CV will be different from the previous one and so you should craft this CV with the new buyers in mind.

Second, make sure you have enough time to spend on your CV. You can't do it if you are being distracted every 2 minutes. Set aside an hour when you aren't going to be disturbed and you have the environment to think about what you want to say and how you are going to sell yourself.

WHAT ARE THE BUYERS IN THE MARKET TO BUY?

With your blank sheet, imagine you are one of the employers who will be reviewing the applications of all the candidates. Write down what they will be looking for. Cluster topics under a number of headings:

- clinical background
- academic performance
- management, leadership and teamworking skills
- personal impact
- teaching and being taught.

If provided, the person specification criteria for the post will help.

Ask the expert
If I don't have one of the essential requirements listed on the person-specification form should I bother applying?
In general, no: you will not be shortlisted. But there are some exceptions, particularly relating to the exact details of previous six-month attachments. If you really want the job, contact one of the consultants directly and ask whether they would consider you.

Once you have finished clustering the lists of what the buyers are in the market to buy, draw maps linking what you can describe in order to satisfy each of these requirements.

This structure gives you the momentum to begin to work out how to lay out the CV and forms the basis of the 'sale' you are trying to make.

PAST PERFORMANCE PREDICTS FUTURE PERFORMANCE

This fundamental headhunter's maxim is true in medicine as well. People who have demonstrated clear, reproducible success for a previous employer will do it for a new employer also. Leopards don't change their spots.

Headhunters use this principle to attract successful people to new jobs. In medicine there aren't any headhunters so you need to do this for yourself.

You want the readers of your CV to be impressed enough with what you have to offer to believe that you can perform when it comes to doing their job.

Top Tip

I repeatedly use the word 'success'. Not every day of every job is positive, and not every experience you have during any given period of time is successful. But it is success and achievement – not experience – that sell you. Whenever you see the word 'experience' substitute 'success'.

AN EXAMPLE OF 'SUCCESS'

Two different SHOs finished exactly the same rotation. One attended outpatients, did ward duties more than competently and functioned as a perfectly good SHO. The other fostered links with the other members of the multiprofessional team, reorganised the outpatient booking process and presented cases at regional grand rounds.

Both had *exactly the same experience* but they are selling completely different things. The second is more likely to get shortlisted. The reason is that the first SHO is simply stating what his or her job description for the post would have been. *It isn't a success simply to do your job.* The second SHO will impress the panel because they will believe that this person will be a successful employee in the future too. The second SHO is much more likely to get the job.

ADDING FLESH TO YOUR ACHIEVEMENTS: POSITIVE POWER VERBS

Read the example again and note the language used to describe the two SHOs. The most active part of English is the verb and it is therefore the verb that is the 'selling' part of the achievement.

The first 'attended' clinic, 'did' duties and 'functioned' competently. All passive words that do not inspire the reader.

The second 'fostered', 'reorganised' and 'presented'. All these verbs are active, positive, exciting and stimulating. They are positive power verbs (PPVs). It is human nature to be more impressed with this language and so using PPVs in your CV will always draw the reader to the activity that it describes.

Positive power verbs

accomplished	built	diagnosed	generated	planned	restored
achieved	chaired	directed	guided	prepared	sampled
advanced	coached	drafted	influenced	presented	scheduled
advised	commenced	enabled	informed	prioritised	set up
appraised	compared	encouraged	initiated	processed	shaped
assembled	completed	engaged	installed	produced	sought
assigned	conducted	established	instigated	programmed	stimulated
assumed	co-ordinated	evaluated	interpreted	promoted	structured
attained	created	expanded	lectured	realised	supervised
audited	critiqued	facilitated	led	recommended	taught
authored	defined	formed	liased	recruited	trained
balanced	designed	formulated	negotiated	remodelled	undertook
began	developed	fostered	organised	researched	validated

If you are finding that you are using the same PPV over and over again, try using the thesaurus function on Word to get some alternatives.

Introducing PPVs

Note that PPVs are always used in the *past tense*. They reflect previous successes and are used to demonstrate the headhunter's maxim that past performance predicts future performance.

PPVs can be introduced in two ways:

> In 2002, I was active in coordinating an audit project into outpatient waiting times. After an initial analysis of the data, we identified weaknesses in the booking process and subsequently implemented changes that improved efficiency and reduced waiting times by an average of 2 weeks.

Or:

> - Coordinated audit of outpatient waiting times, analysed data, implemented changes that resulted in an average reduction in waiting time of 2 weeks.

In the two examples, exactly the same PPVs are used but in different ways. The second example has more impact. First because it is shorter, second because it isn't a sentence – it begins with a bullet point. It is better sales technique to avoid sentences (which have a tendency to require the use of 'I' repeatedly). Begin the sale with a bullet and PPV.

You should use a PPV every time you sell an achievement.

Summary

- In competitive jobs selling your achievements actively to the buyer is vital

- Begin with a blank page, work out what they are likely to want to buy and then map your achievements to these headings

- Sell your achievements with a bullet and a positive power verb

The front page ⬤ 3

In this chapter

- How can you use the front page to stimulate the reader?
- How can you design the front page to be like a newspaper?
- What are your 'big hitters' and how are they skillfully deployed?

The front page of the CV is the most important part. It sets the tone for what is to come and, given that the average CV is read for only 8 seconds, it must follow that *only the front page is read* by many buyers. So the front page is crucial for producing a 'shortlist' decision.

Before you begin to design the front page, go and buy a copy of one of today's newspapers. The front page of a CV and the front page of a newspaper share exactly the same objectives – they both aim to get the reader interested enough to read more. In the case of the paper, the reader then buys the paper; with the CV, the reader shortlists the candidate.

A front cover that simply says 'curriculum vitae' is redundant: the reader knows exactly what it is. If you still aren't persuaded to jettison your front cover, think about all the newspapers you have ever seen: tabloid, broadsheet, small, large, liberal, conservative, colour or black and white. Have you ever seen one with a blank front sheet that simply says, in large letters, 'The Newspaper'? No. Such a thing doesn't exist. The whole point is to stimulate passing readers to look at the front page. If the front page is covered, no-one will have any interest at all in the contents. It is exactly the same for the CV.

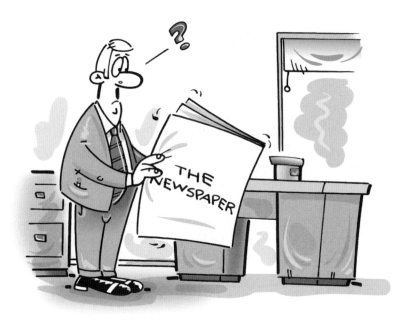

Making the reader want to read more

What are the elements of the newspaper's front page that sell it? First, look at the size of the writing.

TITLE: BRANDING THE REST OF THE PAPER

The title of the paper – *The Times, Daily Express, Guardian* – is always written in the biggest letters. Of course, a lot of newspaper readers buy the same paper every single day of their lives. But even in the paper industry this represents a shrinking percentage as readers become more inquisitive and try out different options. The point is that the editor of the paper wants the readers to remember in *which* paper they found an interesting story or a good columnist. Then they might buy the same paper the next day. They are beginning to develop recognition for the style, taste, views and culture of the paper. The paper is, in other words, developing a brand.

When the buyers read your CV you want them to remember you and recall the contents of your CV when they see you at the interview. This is especially important when you have particular attributes that you want to be brought up at interview.

It is a huge advantage to you at the interview if, among 10 candidates they see, the buyers remember *your* CV. Laying out the CV well and selling your attributes might achieve this. But they have to be able to link the content of your CV easily with your name.

Your name is the only 'brand' you are able to use. You can't call your CV 'superb radiologist for difficult diagnoses'. Your name should be written, just like in the newspaper, in big print in the centre of the top of the front page. You might also consider putting your name on to each subsequent page as a header.

When the readers close the CV before moving on, your name is the last thing they see. This reinforces the information they have read and makes them eager to find out more: by shortlisting you for interview.

Do not ever include a photograph with your CV. It plays to any prejudices your buyers might have (about employing men, or women, or white people, or people with glasses, etc.) and looks unprofessional. You aren't going for a modelling job after all!

HEADLINES

Newspapers also use headlines to great effect. Look at the headlines on your newspaper. Notice the language that is used and the types of words. The words are short and easy to understand. Headlines are snappy, readable at speed and used to entice the reader into continuing to the rest of the article. Even in the broadsheet papers the language used is simple. Editors don't want to introduce words that a percentage of their readers won't understand. A reader would never buy such a paper.

Your CV should be the same: remember that short words are easier to read than long words. It is not a test of your ability to use the dictionary, but a test of your ability to sell your achievements effectively. Buyers want to see whether you are worth shortlisting in the quickest possible time. Don't make it a struggle to understand what you are saying. Say it simply and clearly.

Edit the CV – ask friends to help to ensure this has been achieved. Be ruthless and cut out anything that won't sell you, or is ancient history or is simply wordy and repetitive. You will end up with a much clearer, more saleable result.

Top Tip
Always use short succinct language – make it easy to read for the buyers (including those without a medical background). If there is anything on your CV that an average reader would not necessarily understand, explain it clearly to them. If they don't understand something they are more likely to reject you.

WHICH DIRECTION?

People in the West read in two directions: across from left to right and down from top to bottom. Statistically, different parts of the page are more likely to be read than others. Logically, you should therefore put information that you really want to be read – and that is particularly likely to grab attention – higher up and to the left of the page (see p. 20).

IT'S WHAT YOU DID

It is always what you did that is important. The fact that Crick and Watson won the Nobel prize is more important than the year they made their discovery. Do you even remember which year it was? Why not? Because it doesn't really matter. The fact that they won the prize is more important than the year they won it.

Many CVs have huge lists of every consultant an applicant has ever worked with. It might be flattering to consultants to see their name in print but is that list really adding anything to the sale? Designers of electrical goods don't have their names on the purchase information unless they represent an important part of the brand (like James Dyson). If you must list consultants by name, follow the principles set out in the references chapter (Chapter 5). But remember that the chances of this list selling you are remote.

Top Tip
The principle of ordering information on the CV is what you did on the left, where you did it (and possibly with whom) in the middle, and when on the right.

What → With whom → Where → When

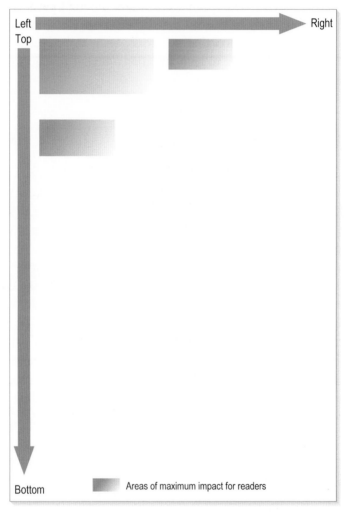

Laying out the page to maximum effect

DATES

A good way to represent the dates you did something is in a single column on the far right of the page. It makes the CV look neat and concise and makes it easy for the reader to ensure there aren't any gaps.

Mind the gap

Professional CV readers spot gaps on CVs from 100 yards. If there are chronological gaps on the CV then make sure you explain what you did with that gap and try to sell that period of your life as an asset. Include times where you were out of medicine to bring up a family or to travel. Otherwise the readers will assume the worst happened in the gap you haven't explained – maybe you were in prison.

TRAILERS

The final lesson from the front page of the newspaper is that trailers can be used as a way of selling content inside the paper to readers. The editor believes these stories or inclusions are so powerful they can simply figure on the front page without further explanation. An exclusive interview with a big star or a new serialisation of a book are examples. Although quite difficult to achieve on a CV, front-page trailers are powerful tools.

BIG HITTERS

This tool is incredibly effective and easy to use.

'Big hitters' is a baseball term. When runners are waiting at first, second or third base, a home run would achieve anything up to four runs. In a game where final scores are usually in single figures, this is hugely significant.

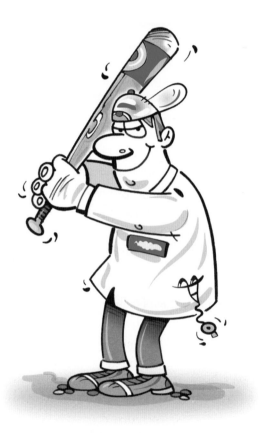

Big hitters

A big hitter is a batsman who can reliably hit a home run in such a situation. The team coach calls out the big hitter to execute the home run and thus score highly.

From the point of view of a CV, a big hitter is anything you have done that would be of such interest to the reader that it would catapult you to the 'shortlist' pile. It doesn't mean things in your past that lots of other people have achieved, but things that are really significant or unique to you.

Big hitters might be related to medicine: like really terrific prizes, or research success or authorship of a seminal book. But they can equally be non-medical. Success in management of a local community event that raised a seven-figure sum for charity would be an example.

When you start writing your CV, define your big hitters. Everyone has some, although it might take a while to think of them and they might well be different between jobs you are applying for. Deploy your big hitters as high up the CV as possible. Definitely on the front page. And as high as you can. This maximises their impact and ensures they are read.

WHAT CAN'T YOU READ?

Return to your newspaper for one last look. On the front page is something that humans cannot read but must be included – the barcode, used when papers are bought in supermarkets to be scanned. Notice where it is placed – the least significant part of the front page. It must be included but has no selling power whatsoever.

The same is true for your personal contact details. Put the information where it is easy to find but make it unimportant in the text. Try placing it immediately below your name but in very small letters. Two or three parallel columns of information usually suffice. Don't make it hard for the Trust to get hold of you.

Give as many contact details as you can. E-mail, mobile, home and work numbers as well as address.

Ask the expert

Do I need to include age, date of birth, place of birth and marital status?

Only date of birth needs to be included. The rest isn't needed. Don't bother about indemnity information. You are applying for a NHS position so this is irrelevant.

A GMC registration number is relevant (and if 'provisional' this should be indicated). If qualifying from outside the UK it is particularly important to make it clear if you have GMC registration.

Summary

- Think of the front page as equivalent to the front page of a newspaper

- Use your name effectively to remind the interviewer of the content of your CV when you return for interview

- Design the CV using short, succinct language throughout

- Find your big hitters and deploy them high up the page and to the left

Employment and education

In this chapter

- How should previous employment and education best be presented?

- How do you 'sell' yourself when describing an examination result or a post held?

- What should you include and what should you leave out?

The backbone of the CV is the record of your previous achievements because past performance is the best predictor of future performance. Your academic results, positions held and other qualifications you hold for the job are vital.

Information packs for prospective job applicants include a table of 'essential' and 'desirable' qualities in applicants. The essential group is most often made up of academic and clinical/research experiences. In simple terms, you cannot apply for an SpR position without passing a postgraduate examination. So make your list of 'essential' attributes clear and easily seen.

WHAT GOES FIRST?

The major principles of ordering the CV are:

- Establish the big hitters as high up as possible.
- Sell the attributes, achievements and experiences the buyers are in the market to buy.
- List everything in reverse chronological order.

With this in mind, employment will usually be stated first. The most relevant element of your past performance is the job you are doing now. Although academic and educational qualifications are important they are not sufficiently distinctive.

 Top Tip
Academic qualifications are not usually distinctive and rarely develop into big hitters. Everyone who is applying for the SpR post must have passed the postgraduate examination. And everyone applying for a Foundation Programme must have passed (or be just about to) MBBS. Although you worked incredibly hard to achieve this success it doesn't help in a competitive field. All it does is level the field. Level fields don't get you jobs.

The exception to this general rule is where you don't have any – or very little – medical employment experience. So for first and second year foundation programmes, current PRHO jobs and first SHO jobs, academic qualifications might take precedence. But for every job after this, always put employment before education.

FIXED AND VARIABLE ACHIEVEMENTS

Accountants use the terms 'fixed costs' and 'variable costs' to describe the inventory of a company and to advise on cost cutting and other financial measures. In the aviation industry, fixed costs would include airport gates, the fleet of planes itself, the head offices and generally the staff employed directly by the company. Variable assets would include beverages and food served to customers, fuel, inflight entertainment, etc.

Fixed costs are defined by their rigidity: thus, short of disposing of an entire aeroplane, it is difficult to vary its cost. Variable costs are more pliable. They can more easily be traded up and down and used to differentiate between competitors. So advertising for different airlines often involves choice of movies, extra leg room, better food, better sleeping accommodation.

When you are listing the various elements of your past you want to include on a CV, it is useful to split them into fixed and variable achievements. Examples are shown below.

Fixed achievements	Variable achievements
Exam results	Presentations
Titles of previous jobs held	Audit work
Prizes won	Positions of responsibility and leadership
Post-graduate qualifications	What you did with the job you held
Medical school attended	Extra-curricular interests
References	Career successes and highlights

The basic principle is that fixed achievements should be stated and variable achievements sold.

For instance, consider the following two lines from the CV of an SHO:

Organised revision programme, accomplished MBBS and negotiated time off to attend graduation ceremony.

And:

Presented paper to regional team meeting on diabetic complications post-surgery; won award for presentation of the year including invitation to speak at national event.

Clearly the first achievement (passing finals) is fixed and to try to sell it in this way is daft. The second is variable and should be sold to demonstrate your personal involvement in the project and how that distinguishes you in the marketplace.

EMPLOYMENT

When you consider your employment history, much of the basic information has to be simply stated. It is fixed. So how can you sell it?

When you ask consultants about SHOs or SpRs they have worked with in the past they clearly differentiate between individuals. Many they remember by name and still keep in touch with. Others are forgotten and (hopefully) won't come asking for a reference because it would be difficult to find much good to say about them.

But all of these previous staff did their jobs. None bunked work, or were incompetent or even rude. The difference between the two groups was what they did with the jobs.

The first group threw themselves into the opportunities provided. They sought research projects, solved problems, taught medical students, built relationships across the multiprofessional environment. Patients liked them. The second group followed the job description down to the last letter and made nothing of the job. They left the post simply with a tick in a box.

The comparison between these two extremes is the key to selling employment achievements. You have to consider what you did that *the average holder of the post would not have done*. Name the job and then use bullet points and PPVs to sell what you believe put you into the first category employees.

 If a buyer wants to read a job description he or she can phone medical staffing to get one. Don't try to sell the job description to the reader. Think what you achieved over and above what most holders of the post would have done, then sell it.

List the jobs according to what you did, where (and possibly with whom) you did it, and then put the dates on the right. Place your previous jobs in reverse chronological order. Don't oversell the case. If you have done more than two different jobs then cluster bullets together under a separate section called 'key achievements'. Don't repeat the same thing for more than one job (e.g. 'set up rota for on-call arrangements'): instead think of different skills under different headings.

Example

Senior House Officer in Endocrinology, Poole Hospitals NHS Trust, 2004/5:

1. Established weekly objective-based teaching for third year medical students.
2. Reviewed management plans at multiprofessional team meetings.
3. Facilitated medical involvement in review of outpatient catering services.
4. Revised cover arrangements compliant with Working Time requirements.
5. Developed skills in lumbar puncture and fundoscopy.

Notice how these points reflect different aspects of your career, which can perhaps be summarised broadly as:

- clinical (bullet 5)
- managerial and leadership (bullet 4)
- academic (bullet 1)
- patient focused (bullet 3)
- teamworking, building relationships and collaboration (bullet 2).

The order is not important but a common mistake is for all the bullets to be based narrowly on clinical achievements. Recognise that developing a great career in medicine involves a multitude of competencies and transferable skills. In a tough field, clinical achievements alone won't get you the job.

ADVANCED SELLING

The best way of selling your achievements is to judge their outcomes. An achievement is impressive on its own but you can be more effective in communicating your skills to the readers if you can relate your achievement to an outcome. You might have raised £5000 by running the London marathon for charity. That's the achievement. The fact that the money was used to buy 100 wheelchairs for use in schools in Scotland is the outcome of your achievement.

It takes time to get this right. People often tell me they don't know what the outcome of their achievement was. What happened as a result of their audit project, or whether the new rota they composed worked out or not. Usually there is no reason why the answers cannot be found. And if you can establish that your audit project eventually resulted in reduced waiting list times it makes a much more powerful sell.

LINKING JOBS TOGETHER

One of the reasons for CVs being too long is that lists of jobs (and all 82 consultants you worked with in each job) go on for pages and pages. This isn't selling you, because in battling through all these pages the reader struggles to find your big hitters.

Deal with this by clustering jobs together. Where they formed a rotation call it the 'South East London Rotation' and then sell your achievements as above. Avoid long lists of consultants and remember you don't need lots of space between jobs: put them on consecutive lines to keep brief.

EDUCATION

Educational achievements are even harder to sell. They are all fixed achievements, all 'essential' for the position. Despite the personal struggle to achieve the qualifications (from school upwards) they are very poor discriminators in competitive fields. This is particularly true at earlier stages in the medical career.

Later on, research posts, higher qualifications (Masters, PhDs, MDs etc.) become significant because not all the candidates will possess one. At SpR interview level and above it is one extra point that you might be able to use to your advantage. If this is the case, all associated achievements should be listed (such as presentations, especially to key international conferences, papers and research symposia).

Ask the expert
How far back do I need to go with academic qualifications? This depends very much on how strong 'ancient history' results were. Strong all-A performances at GCSE and A levels would remain on the CV for some years afterwards. But the fact you got a B in History at GCSE when you are going for a clinical director role in your mid-40s is not relevant. So it is a balance between suggesting a solid track-record of academic performance and judging the relevance of the qualification to the application. Academic performance at age 16 certainly suggests that strong academic performance is likely in the future but if there is no success in the meantime, good grades at age 16 are negated.

HOW TO SELL EDUCATIONAL QUALIFICATIONS

The key is to link the qualification to other achievements that others with the same paper results may not have. In Chapter 5, publications, presentations and audits will be considered in full as these generally go on the second page. But you might have a big hitter as part of an academic portfolio. Academic big hitters might include:

- first-class honours or distinctions at any level
- prize-level performances at finals
- winning a competition or prize
- achieving a specific level of funding or sponsorship for research from an internationally known source
- presenting research or data at a key international event
- genuine breakthrough data or unexpectedly strong results.

Where you can link a big hitter to the academic qualification, you should do so. Otherwise treat all educational qualifications as being fixed achievements and simply state them. As always, present them in reverse chronological order, state what you achieved on the left and the date you achieved it on the right.

 Top Tip
Any awards and prizes should be treated as big hitters and brought forward, stated on the left hand side of the page and as far up as possible.

Summary

- Unless this is your first or second job in medicine, always place employment before educational qualifications

- Don't attempt to restate job descriptions but think of ways of selling your 'overachievement' in a post

- What did you achieve that the average holder of the post would not have done?

- Look for big hitters in your education and sell them strongly

Adding depth to the CV: the second page

5

In this chapter

- What additional features about your career should you include?
- How can these be used to increase your chances of being shortlisted?
- What is the best way of bringing in references and outside interests?

The CV should be as short as possible. The longer it is, the less likely it will be read. Page 2 is less likely to be read than page 1, page 3 less than page 2, etc. Be brutal and edit your CV to be as short as possible, without letting go of the fundamental need for it to effectively sell your successes.

There are no rules about the ordering of information on the CV, although it would be very strange to put your charitable work and position as a captain of a local amateur sports team as the first item. Employment and education are usually listed first, after that you decide on what follows.

 Don't use too many headings and subheadings: they have no impact in selling your achievements. Avoid using more than four headings per page and remove subheadings altogether. For instance don't put 'Interests' as the heading and then add superfluous subheadings like 'Sporting', 'Charitable', 'Musical', etc. Simply list the interests in whatever order is most effective in selling to the reader.

TRANSFERABLE SKILLS

A really effective second page involves transferable skills that would be listed for a non-medical job application, and many would appear on a CV of someone in a different profession. You are trying to paint a picture of a competent, successful person in life and showing a track record of achievement.

Headings to consider

Chapter 4 defined several clusters of employment-related skills. Including as many of these as possible is a very strong way of selling. These headings were:

- clinical
- managerial and leadership
- academic
- patient focused
- teamworking, relationship building, multiprofessional working.

A really good candidate can describe all of these skills: they define what makes an effective doctor and builds a great career in medicine. Decide what to include by considering each of these headings again.

MANAGEMENT AND LEADERSHIP

Demonstrating an understanding of the importance of management is a huge boost to a CV. 'Management skills' is probably the most overused buzzword in the whole of the application process, but includes three basic themes:

- self-motivation and discipline, including time management
- managing teams, particularly in a multiprofessional setting
- managing organisations and influencing their strategic direction.

Demonstrating these is difficult: this is the hardest section of the CV to get right. It has the potential to sound trite and affected. It is also the easiest section in which to massively exaggerate your experiences. After all, running an amateur dramatic society really isn't the same as being Chief Executive of an NHS Trust.

The trick is to consider what you have done that would be considered management and then to sell that in a measured, effective way.

In the first few years of a medical career these skills will come from outside the field of employment. They might relate to university activities or extracurricular life. Management ability is measured by outcomes. So work on the advanced selling described in Chapter 4. Work out what the achievement is you are trying to describe and then find the outcome of that achievement. If you are using captaincy of a sports team then what did the team accomplish while you were in charge? If it is committee work, how did that benefit the people you were supposed to be representing?

Top Tip
If you can get the concept that you were 'elected' to a position into the CV that is extremely effective. It is a simple word that says a lot. It implies that other people like you, or at least trust you enough to represent them. It says you are a team player.

ACADEMIC BACKGROUND

There will always be more to this than simply postgraduate examinations, medical school performance and school grades. Some of the additional achievements you could list here are big hitters and should be included on the front page. But others will add depth to your CV and personality and can neatly be packaged further down. Five aspects are included:

- grades and formal qualifications (already considered)
- academic publications (books and papers)
- presentations
- prizes and awards
- clinical governance.

ACADEMIC PUBLICATIONS

Papers are fixed attributes and should be listed and not sold. We all know that a paper in the *Lancet* is more impressive than the local community newsletter, and peer-reviewed papers are always superior.

The way you cite references is arbitrary but must be consistent. People obsess about whether you should adopt the '*BMJ* style' or '*NEJM* style'. Honestly, it doesn't matter. Decide on how you want to cite your papers and refer to each of them the same way. Put them in reverse chronological order.

Include the title of the paper, journal, volume number, page numbers and year. Many people list all the authors of the paper on their CV but this isn't necessary and can take up a huge amount of non-selling space. If you are citing the paper it is obvious that you are one of the authors. And you aren't there to sell the other authors, they can quite happily sell themselves.

 Buyers see right through tricks like listing several papers that are in progress. You should avoid this. First, it tends to dent the significance of the ones that are complete. And second, your CV is a record of past achievement and not a crystal ball. Those papers might never be completed, let alone accepted. Leave them out.

Book credits should also be listed here. These are stronger than papers as fewer applicants will have them. You should, therefore, try to consider these as variable achievements and sell your involvement using bullets and PPVs. For example:

- Developed concept for new combination book and CD-ROM on heart sounds, identified contributors and published book with Poole Publishing.

The name of the publisher should be included.

 Top Tip
There is no doubt that a really solid list of papers is an advantage on a CV. If you have lots of papers to list, don't fill pages and pages here but add the list as a bibliography at the end. And remember, if you don't want to include every single paper you have ever written, you don't have to.

PRESENTATIONS

Early on in a medical career these are a very useful achievement to sell. PRHOs and early-stage SHOs, and definitely medical students, rarely get the chance to present formally. It tends to be people with the most get-up-and-go that push themselves forward into the few opportunities that exist. So at this stage in the career, presentations are big hitters that should be sold strongly. The bigger the audience and the less local the meeting, the better.

Examples include:

- hospital grand rounds
- major audit or clinical governance meetings
- any regional or national meetings
- any meetings where key aspects of research were presented (e.g. following a BSc project)
- lectures, such as to the entire medical school.

PRIZES AND AWARDS

Not everyone has won a prize and not all prizes are worth winning, let alone naming on a CV. Remember, it isn't how hard you worked to get something that matters. What is important is the impression that listing the achievement on the CV makes on the reader.

Some prizes, like major university awards, might be big hitters and should definitely be pushed up to the front page. And if prizes link directly to qualifications they should be listed immediately following the qualification.

Top Tip
Don't go back to previous items listed on your CV. If you are describing a qualification, sell the prizes that you won at the same time as receiving the qualification immediately. It tends to make readers sea-sick if they have to keep referring back to something.

If relevant, non-medical prizes can also be listed.

It is easy to demolish the effectiveness of selling something really strong by attaching it to something weak:

● First prize, Medical Division, University of London 2002
● Prize for best improver, Poole Junior Swimming Club 1987

CLINICAL GOVERNANCE

One of the most important developments in the last decade has been the introduction of clinical governance. Including continuous professional development, quality assurance and audit, clinical

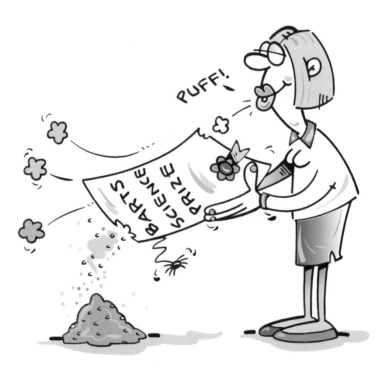

'Ah, here it is . . .'

governance is designed to make the profession more self-critical and evidence based. You should try to get some examples onto your CV, showing that you understand the principles of clinical governance and that your own practice abides by its framework.

PATIENT FOCUSED

One of the most depressing parts of the medical selection process is that patients tend to be forgotten. Over the next 5 to 10 years, selection will change to include some sort of assessment of applicants' abilities to relate to patients.

Because it isn't formally assessed, it is a huge boost to your CV if you can introduce elements where you have proved an ability to represent or work with patients towards a common goal. These are the least frequent skills quoted and therefore the most powerful.

In Trusts, it tends to be nurses who act on committees looking at patients' interests. But there is no reason why this should be the case. Artwork on the walls, refreshments that are provided, transport links to outpatients, translator services and openness of access to visitors are all areas where there might be a hospital committee. In preparing yourself for future application processes, consider how you might get involved with patients in your current hospital.

If you can include patient-related activities on your CV somewhere, make sure you emphasise what the patients got out of your involvement.

TEAMWORKING, RELATIONSHIP BUILDING AND MULTIPROFESSIONAL WORK

All doctors need to be able to do all three of these. Try to find some examples where you have shown an ability to network, work collaboratively towards common ends, and across a broad spectrum of professional and non-professional interests. This section will most likely be drawn from non-medical activities. This is discussed in Chapter 9.

THE END OF THE CV: INTERESTS AND REFERENCES

It is traditional, but not essential, to include your interests on a CV. In practically every other field of life references are not included on the CV but are taken up after you are offered a position. Unfortunately, in medicine it would be considered strange if you did not include references.

Interests

The basic principles for describing your interests are:

- Be truthful (don't say you like Shakespeare if you have never read or seen one of his plays).
- Keep the interests in perspective (don't say you competed for Britain in tennis if you mean you supervise your children in tennis lessons on Saturday mornings).
- Don't try too hard (just because you don't run marathons every 6 weeks doesn't make you a bad person).
- Don't list too many (begs the question as to whether you ever do any work).

But otherwise don't obsess about this section: it will hardly be noticed unless you share an interest with one of the buyers (in which case it might be something they will bring up at interview and thus a potential asset).

References

Choosing references

It is at best highly inappropriate and at worse discriminatory for doctors to be expected to provide references before the selection process actually begins. Are the names of the references being used to endorse your application? Well, yes. So in this case it is good advice to get the biggest 'names' in the field to act as your reference.

On the other hand, the reference needs to know you and remember who you are. So getting someone who knows you better – and isn't a big 'name' – is more likely to produce a personalised, honest reference.

Choosing who to ask is an art in itself. But there should never be more than three. This means jettisoning references as you move through your career. One of the references should be from your current employer. They don't all have to be from doctors: hospital managers and other leaders can provide references. But they are professionally supplied, meaning that personal friends or contacts from outside the NHS should not normally be used.

Listing references
Always put the references in alphabetical order and be completely consistent in how you state them:

Dr John P Smith	Dr S Jones
Consultant Cardiologist & Head of Clinical Research Unit	Adam Hospitals NHS Trust Adam, AD1 1DA
Poole Hospitals NHS Trust	Switchboard: 020 1000 1000
Poole, PO1 1OP	
Direct tel: 020 0000 0000	
Mobile: 07900 000000	
E-mail: smith@poole.nhs.uk	

The problem with the example above is that it implies you know the first person better (because you supply his first name and both mobile phone and e-mail address) and you respect him more (because you put him first despite his being S to the other reference's J, and you use his title).

The format does not matter but you must be consistent. So if you provide one e-mail address you must provide all of them; if you use one first name, use all of their first names. As with your own personal details (see Chapter 3), you should make it easy for the employing hospital to contact the references. Provide as many contact routes as you can.

Summary

- Be ruthless in what to include and what to edit out of the second part of the CV

- Keep in mind the buyers and what they are likely to be interested in

- Where possible, include examples that involve patient or community work, teamworking, relationship building and management

- Never be tempted to over-egg the cake and ensure that everything you write is believable

- Interests and references should be stated simply and clearly at the end

Researching application forms

6

In this chapter

- How do you obtain an application form?

- What are the most commonly asked questions?

- Are there any patterns that apply to the content of forms for different grades of jobs?

Identifying trends and patterns in application forms will better enable you to prepare answers that will increase your chances of success.

In researching this book, a project was undertaken to review job advertisements in *BMJ Careers* between August 2003 and July 2004 over several discrete weeks. The results of this extensive analysis are detailed below.

SCOPE OF RESEARCH

Applications were made for 200 substantive UK-based posts between SHO and Consultant level. Positions not included in the research were PRHO, staff- and Trust-grade positions, associate specialist posts and locum jobs.

1. Grades

Position applied for	Number of applications
Consultant	49
SpR	20
Research position	36
SHO	91

Every specialty was included. Initial analysis of application forms indicated marked differences by Trusts in requirements for SHO and higher levels, so SpR, consultant and research jobs are grouped together for analysis.

2. Geography

Furthest application	NHS Trust
Furthest North application	Highland NHS Trust
Furthest South application	Jersey NHS Trust
Furthest West application	Cornwall Primary Care Trust
Furthest East application	East Essex NHS Trust

OBTAINING THE FORMS: WRITTEN ADVERTISEMENTS AND INTERNET VERSIONS

At present, medical jobs are advertised by the Trust that is offering the post. *BMJ Careers* and certain other publications (such as college or specialty journals) also contain job listings. *BMJ Careers* advertises 95% of all available medical jobs.

The internet also contains a huge number of medical job portals that are regularly updated. This is not the only means of finding a job, but it is the quickest. In addition, the NHS is developing a website that combines all this information, but this is not available at time of going to press. *BMJ Careers* currently publishes all its advertised jobs online.

Different Trusts require your application to be made in totally different ways. There is no obvious pattern to the process between Trusts. But single Trusts seem to use the same style of application for all available jobs, at all grades and for all specialties.

The contrasting ways of obtaining an application pack can be summarised as:

- telephoning medical personnel to ask for the required documents to be posted
- e-mail-based application: request documents by post or via the internet
- downloading the application form from the Trust's website.

Telephoning the Trust

One third of the posts applied for were available only by phone. Some Trusts have people to talk to and others use a 24-hour answerphone. Expect a delay of 5 days before receiving the pack. Every single form was delivered within this period. A sizeable portion of the Amazon rainforest is sure to arrive on your doormat – the heaviest application pack (from Leeds Mental Health NHS Trust) cost £2.36 in postage.

E-mail-based application

Many hospitals offer an e-mail return service that sends forms to individual applicants' e-mail addresses. All of our e-mails were replied to within 24 hours of application or packs were delivered promptly by post. There was one exception – Eastern Deanery – who finally replied to an application request after 7 days.

Downloaded forms

Many Trusts have the application form, job description, person specification and possibly a local map on their websites. This is by far the fastest way to obtain the information. Some also have the facility to deal with completed and returned forms electronically.

> **Top Tip**
> Many Trusts do not include the name of the job for which you have applied in the information. If, like us, you 'applied' for over 200 jobs you should keep a list of what you have applied for and manage the downloaded forms carefully. You might otherwise accidentally apply for the wrong job at the wrong hospital.

TIME TO CLOSING DATE

Irrespective of the delivery method used, there was no difference in the length of time to closing dates for applications.

APPLICATION BY CV

26% of posts accepted application by CV only.

How many CVs and how many copies?

The graph at the top of p. 48 splits all the positions we examined into: SHO posts, and combined SpR, research and consultant posts. It illustrates the average number of copies of CVs that were required for application, the maximum number asked for by any recruiting Trust, and the number of Trusts where no CV is required.

Fewer CVs were requested for SHO posts.

> **Top Tip**
> Always send a CV even if they discourage it, because *your* CV is always a better sales tool than *their* application form.

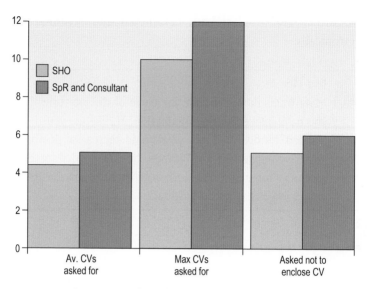

Average number of copies of CVs expected

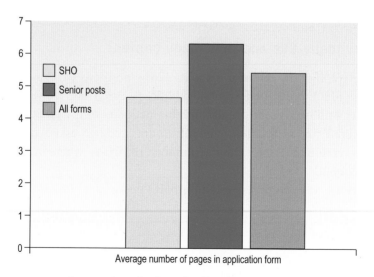

Average length of application form (in pages)

TYPICAL APPLICATION FORMS

The forms varied greatly in length from two to fourteen sides (A4), with the average length for all posts looked at being 5.5 sides. Application forms for SHO appointments were shorter (on average) than for senior positions (see below).

Only 5% of the forms were specifically created for the job advertised. In other words, most were generic and applied to all medical jobs offered within the Trust at all grades.

WHAT ARE THE DIFFERENT SUBSECTIONS OF APPLICATION FORMS?

All the questions on all application forms can be divided into two types (see Chapter 7):

- fixed questions
- variable questions.

Fixed questions

These questions require a simple answer. They include:

- contact details
- employment record
- a list of your qualifications and where they were obtained
- a list of prizes and other awards
- the name of your current post.

Variable questions

These questions require crafted responses – they provide an opportunity to sell your achievements. Questions asked on application forms can be classified into one of five categories:

- academic background
- clinical experience and achievements

- teaching
- management
- personal criteria.

Each of the questions listed is considered in detail in Chapter 9.

1. Academic questions
Asked about in:

- 19 % of SHO forms
- 36% of Senior forms.

The most common categories of question were:

Question	Number of forms containing question
1. Courses attended	45
2. Research, posters and presentation achievements	43
3. Prizes and distinctions in career to date	39
4. Membership of a learned body	31

2. Clinical experience
Asked about in:

- 11% of SHO forms
- 36% of Senior forms.

Specific questions covered experience, audit and training. A few Trusts were interested in specific lists of procedures performed (5%). The same proportion found IT skills of interest. The top 5 questions asked in our sample are shown below:

1. What clinical experience do you have?	37
2. Audit experience	23
3. Provide details of your clinical training	21
4. Procedures and ability	19
5. Describe your clinical duties	12

3. Teaching
Asked about in:

- 10% of SHO forms
- 33% of Senior forms.

Top Tip
Forms also used the terms 'aptitude' and 'training', which should be taken to mean the same as achievements to provide a model answer that can be replicated for different jobs you are applying for.

4. Management
Asked about in:

- 3% of SHO forms
- 12% of Senior forms.

1. Teamwork experience (multidisciplinary team)	9
2. Leadership experience	8
3. Communication skills	8

5. Personal criteria
Asked about in:

- 21% of SHO forms
- 47% of Senior forms.

This section provides your best chance to sell yourself on the form. Sometimes, answers are word-capped but, on the other hand, one-quarter of the posts encouraged the use of additional sheets where needed.

The most common questions were:

1. Provide a personal statement in support of your application	51
2. The JFK question (see Chapter 15)	37
3. Can you drive?	28
4. What is your current salary?	26
5. Why are you leaving your current job?	25
6. Time off work for illness	24
7. When can you start the job?	18

The application form 'Hall of Fame and Shame'

Most incompetent department: application form not included in posted pack	Sherwood Forest NHS Trust
Daftest question: 'Please note in order to comply with our Equal Opportunities Policy, if you are submitting a CV please <u>do not</u> (their underlining) include any personal details.'	Leeds Teaching Hospitals NHS Trust
Second daftest question: 'We strongly advise candidates against providing false data when applying.'	East Sussex NHS Trust
Most offensive looking form: mint green paper	Milton Keynes NHS Trust
Most frustrating application: 11 phone calls to get a pack sent out!	Liverpool Women's Health Hospital NHS Trust
Slowest response: 7 days to reply to an e-mail request for application details	Eastern Deanery

Admitting defeat: the Royal Marsden NHS Trust sent a letter withdrawing an advertised post but with no contact details so we could not follow-up the reasons for this bizarre waste of time and NHS resources

Hall of fame: star award for most lavish pack:	Papworth NHS Trust
● Multi-coloured, Velcro flip tab outer folder entitled 'Are you a Papworth person?' ● Neatly produced, hand-signed, personalised letter ● Coffee-proof application form ● Map booklet with four maps of location ● Full-colour copy of the hospital's annual report, called 'Climbing mountains together'	

Summary

● This research has shown contrasting quantity and quality of information provided with applications

● The format, style and length of application forms are not consistent

● The research identifies the most common application form questions, which are considered in detail in Chapter 9

Introduction to application forms and the link to the CV

7

In this chapter

- Why are application forms used?
- How should you begin to prepare for the completion of application forms?
- What are the potential time-savers in their completion?

The two-stage model for success in medical job applications is

CV/application form → Shortlisted for interview → Job offer

Many Trusts (although not all – see Chapter 6) have introduced a further hurdle: as well as producing a CV, an application form must be completed. If provided, an assessment of this form is part of the shortlisting criteria.

Application forms are bad for the candidate and good for the recruiters. The reasons for this are:

- Application forms are almost always generic, i.e. not specific for the job you are applying for, whereas the CV should always be designed to be job specific.
- Questions can be asked on an application form which cover areas in which you don't have any specific experience: there is therefore the risk that you will have to leave blank spaces.
- They tend to encourage you to waffle, rather than sell your achievements succinctly.

● You still have to prepare a CV, creating more work. When the process involves both a CV and application form, it is longer and more tedious.

NEGATIVE EXPERIENCE

All of this tends to create a feeling of doom around the job application process. Sometimes it feels like the minute you have arrived in one job you need to begin applying for the next.

In other walks of life, moving jobs is less frequent and less time consuming. Because you, the employee, have made a decision to look around for a new opportunity, it tends to be a positive experience. I don't know of any other job for which you are asked to supply up to 12 copies of the CV and application form.

OVER APPLYING

There is also a culture of 'over applying', which has two direct consequences. First, the work involved is multiplied. Many doctors apply for 10 or more jobs, with the inevitable time-consuming, concentrated administration. And this also results in a kind of 'catch-all' CV and application form being created and used for each one.

A 'standard' CV ignores the sales premise, which is that you have to find out what the buyer wants and then sell into those requirements. Different Trusts have different needs and in preparing a common CV you decrease your chances of success by lack of focus.

Overapplying also causes the recruiting Trusts to worry that a good candidate won't take a job even if offered. Frequently, you are asked to tell the panel the same afternoon as the interview whether you are taking the job, and you will be bound by this. You don't even have the chance to discuss it with partner or family in a situation where a house move will be required. But with the 'over apply' culture you can understand the reasons why the Trusts make this demand.

OPENING THE APPLICATION FORM

 Never forget to sell yourself: don't be trapped by the wording of the form into bland, passive, boring prose.

Our analysis of the application process confirms that questions fall into one of two categories, represented by fixed and variable achievements. Fixed achievements are those that are simply facts recorded as data, or dates or letters. Variable achievements require explanation. Fixed achievements are stated and variable achievements sold.

Fixed attributes often represent half of all the questions on the form and can be dealt with very quickly, as they will simply be stated.

 Top Tip
When you first start to fill in forms, photocopy them and cut out every question so they appear separately. Divide the piles into the fixed and variable styles. Then fill in the fixed pile straight away. All of a sudden the opportunities for sales become much more obvious, and much more manageable.

Reduce the amount of work by repeating sections of your CV. When you consider the whole list of questions asked (the most common are described in detail in Chapter 9) there is a good chance that many of them will already feature on the CV. Don't worry about repeating yourself, remember you want the recruiters to see and remember your big hitters and so the more they see them the better.

Summary

- The introduction of an application form is bad for the candidate

- Application forms can often encourage you to stop selling yourself

- At the outset, work out which of the questions are about fixed attributes (these are just stated) and which are about variable attributes – these should be sold

8

Filling in the application form

In this chapter

- How do you begin filling in the application form?

- How do you sell yourself effectively using the application form?

- What clues are given in the form about the evaluation criteria used for the job?

SAVING TIME

Don't procrastinate. When you have received the application form complete it on one or at most two attempts. Begin with the fixed achievements and simply fill in the answers to these questions. This completes half of the form, and sometimes even more.

Don't leave the form on the kitchen table waiting to be completed. Instead use the simple, effective rule of time management, which is only to 'touch' every piece of paper that comes across your desk once. In other words, in one action you transfer the piece of paper from the in-tray to the out-tray.

More importantly, don't take the paperwork into the mess and try to complete it there. You don't want your colleagues to know what you are applying for, and you certainly don't want their opinions on how to fill in the forms.

As far as the CV is concerned, it is helpful to have opinions from others as to the style and content you have put together. But the application form is one big trap, and it is likely that your colleagues have already fallen into it. The forms are designed to try to level a competitive playing field and it is a harder sell for the candidates using the application form. Your 'advisers' have probably fallen into the trap and their advice is likely to be counterproductive for you.

PRINCIPLES OF SELLING USING APPLICATION FORMS

The reason why I refer to the application form as a trap is that it actively discourages selling. But selling is the best way to get shortlisted and you have to remember that a level playing field never helps candidates, especially in a competitive job market. Any opportunity you have to sell your achievements should be grasped.

Remember, you are only selling the variable achievements. Fixed achievements are simply stated. Less than half the form will allow a sales opportunity so ensure you use *every single one* of the available 'variable achievements' questions.

The basic principles of selling using the application form are:

- Type the form if possible.
- Remember that we read left to right and top to bottom, so get the most important part of the information you want to convey to the top left of the box provided.
- Place all dates in reverse chronological order, unless specifically asked not to.
- Don't be tempted to write in sentences.

The application form tempts you to forget the basic tenet of the CV, which is never to use a sentence. Bullets and PPVs are much better sales weapons.

- Use a bullet followed by a positive power verb.
- The outcomes of the achievements are always the most important part.
- What you achieved is most important, followed by where, followed by when: put the dates on the right hand side of the page.
- Get your big hitters in at every opportunity.
- Keep the points succinct; don't worry about not filling every centimetre of the box.

> Often, the boxes provided are too big. If you try to fill in all the allocated space you will waffle, reducing the impact of the answer. Leave some blank space in the box to make information easier to read even if it is typed. Edit the boxes and ensure you have only included information that will effectively sell. No waffle.

- And finally, don't forget that any opportunity to refer to and trailer other aspects of your career (which might be detailed on the CV) should be taken: you *want* the reader to look at your CV as well: it is a much better sales aid.

MULTIPLE APPLICATIONS

If you are applying for different jobs at the same time, the CV should be tailored for each job individually. This is particularly important in rotations where different specialties are offered, and at different types of hospital. What is relevant for a professorial post at a teaching hospital might not be quite the same as a busy clinical job at a DGH, for instance.

Application forms for different posts vary enormously. If the form seems to be specific for the post, rather than generic for all jobs the Trust is advertising, it will need more time. On the other hand, some forms are just lists of fixed achievement questions, which take little time to complete.

You might be able to complete lots of forms the same day, to save time, but be careful to send all the information back to the right HR department!

INTRODUCING BIG HITTERS

One of the most frequent questions I am asked is how to bring big hitters into the application form. Big hitters are successes that stand out and are most likely to result in being shortlisted. They should also be used as extensively as possible in the interview. It is to your advantage to make sure that you have introduced all of your big hitters and used them effectively.

The problem is that you might not be able to introduce some or all of your big hitters.

There is a balance between the need to sell your big hitters and not listing achievements that aren't relevant to the question being asked. In this latter case you might not be able to mention the specific achievement in the form.

That's why you always include your CV. Even if they are not using it strictly as part of the selection criteria, your big hitters will be prominently and effectively sold. Glancing through a CV when supplied is human nature and if a shortlister sees a big hitter there, it might be enough to call you to interview.

BEING POSITIVE: WHAT ARE THE BENEFITS OF THE APPLICATION FORM TO THE JOB SEEKER?

There are two advantages to the candidate when an application form is used:

- greater use of non-medical achievements
- insight into the potential selection criteria for the post.

Non-medical achievements

Unlike the CV, where these tend to be pushed to the end and down-played, some of the application forms pick non-medical achievements out and build them up.

This is an advantage to the applicant. Such activities suggest a breadth of character and an ability to work with people or in a team, and someone with whom the shortlister might enjoy working. They are also easier to sell and never sound arrogant. So always take opportunities to detail your non-career successes.

How can you use the application form to work out the selection criteria for the job?

Some information packs include a list of selection criteria, or a person specification. This is usually broken down into essential and desirable characteristics. Our analysis indicated that this was infrequent for SHO jobs. When jobs were CV-only, a selection criteria list was never included.

Top Tip
Don't be too worried if you seem not to have that many of the 'desirable' characteristics that are listed. Very few candidates will have the entire list. It is often an advantage not to have so many because it implies you are younger, up-and-coming and therefore attractive to the employer.

In addition, if specific questions on management, academic success, teamworking, etc. are deployed it is likely that one of the 'points' for the selection will be gained by answering that question. And if the form seems to have been created as a catch-all for every available job some of the questions will be more relevant than others.

YOUR OWN HANDWRITING

There is frequently a section where you are asked to complete the answer in your own writing. Many people in medicine feel embarrassed about their handwriting. I'm never sure where this idea that one answer should be hand-written has come from, but if a section is included:

- write it yourself: asking a friend is at best dishonest and at worse fraudulent
- take your time, especially if you think your handwriting is a problem
- write in black.

EXTRA PAGES

In our survey, candidates for a third of all senior jobs were encouraged to use extra sheets of paper. This is another application form trap because it is tempting to fill the entire sheet. The succinct sales bullets of the CV turn into sentence-bound waffle.

The one exception to falling into this trap is where you have a large list of papers that need to be quoted. Add a bibliography to the CV and reference that on the form. Apart from anything else, this strategy will get your CV looked at.

Summary

- Be efficient about completing the form and give yourself enough time
- Work out what you are going to sell (the variable achievements) and then sell these in exactly the same way as in the CV
- Avoid using extra sheets and leave space on the form to allow readability

9

Top 20 application form questions

In this chapter

- What are the 20 most common questions on application forms?
- How should you prepare the answers to these?
- Where are the opportunities to sell your achievements in these answers?

In drawing up a list of the most commonly used questions on application forms, all the fixed achievement questions (name, qualifications, contact details, employment record, references, etc.) have been excluded.

Where questions are similarly posed and have the same meaning they are listed together, for example:

- Why do you want the job?
- What makes you best qualified for the job?
- Why should you be considered for the job?

ACADEMIC BACKGROUND

Question	Percentage of forms that asked question
1. Which courses have you attended?	45
2. Research, posters and presentation achievements?	43
3. Prizes and distinctions in career to date?	39
4. Membership of a learned body?	31

Courses attended

This was a surprisingly common question in this group. The principles when answering it are to:

- Ensure courses are recent and relevant.
- Identify any with competitive entry criteria (e.g. 100 applied for 10 places).
- Don't include courses that are ancient history.
- Highlight courses where you won a prize or best improver, etc.
- Don't include non-career courses here (swimming instructor's course, music examiner's course, etc.).

Research, posters and presentations

- List papers as described for the CV and don't worry which 'style' (*BMJ*, *Lancet*, etc.) you use – so long as it is consistent throughout the list.
- If the list is very long, append a bibliography to the CV and refer to that.
- Presentations should be included if:
  - they have been made to a respected international audience
  - they relate to a specific piece of research and especially to BSc, MD and PhD dissertations
  - you are going for PRHO and SHO posts and they are at least hospital, or medical-school-wide.
- The reader might not know what your research is about and extra explanation might be required.

Prizes and distinctions

Many completed application forms will not have anything in this box. Don't make up awards. Ensure what you write is credible.

- Don't mention school prizes unless they really are big hitters.
- If the readers won't understand what a prize is for, explain it to them.
- If the prize is a real achievement then sell it hard.

Membership of a learned body

This was the biggest surprise in the top 20. First, because there isn't really a list of what constitutes a 'learned body' and second because membership can be awarded based on all sorts of criteria, including a hefty wallet.

- If possible, try to link membership with specific outcomes: what have you done with the membership.
- If you aren't in a learned body then don't put anything down.
- Royal Colleges and memberships of subspecialty groups would probably be included but the BMA would not (it's a union).

CLINICAL EXPERIENCE AND ACHIEVEMENTS

Question	Percentage of forms that asked question
1. What clinical experience do you have?	37
2. Audit experience	23
3. Provide details of your clinical training	21
4. Procedures and ability	19
5. Describe your clinical duties	12

What clinical experience do you have?

It is really important not to recite your job description. One of two traps (see Duties, below), this question can be misunderstood and answered by listing your daily routine. Instead, demonstrate to the reader how you were *better* than the average holder of your post(s).

- Cluster jobs together to avoid repetition.
- Think of some good subheadings under which to group achievements.
- If management, teamwork, etc. are not asked about elsewhere on the form you should include any achievements under these headings here too.
- Don't bore the readers to death.

Audit experience

Everybody has been involved in audit. The problem is that a lot of audit is a complete waste of time. Audit involves a cycle of activity: it isn't just about doing some sort of survey. Experienced assessors of application forms can easily judge the quality of your audit project.

- Include only genuine audit (with clear outcomes).
- Demonstrate what the audit achieved, i.e. not just an analysis of waiting times but an action plan to reduce them and a review of progress.
- Emphasise what the audit did for patients.
- Make it clear you played an active part (with the use of PPVs) (see Chapter 2).

Details of clinical training

Similar to the first question but subtly different. This question is more about the training you have received to be ready for the job you are now applying for rather than the experiences you can describe. Where possible, you should discuss training plans, appraisal and objectives that have been set together with

educational supervisers to demonstrate that you have kept up with
what has been agreed.

- Do not write about educational achievements (like degrees).
- Again, you might be able to introduce a big hitter that doesn't
  fit anywhere else.
- This question does not ask for a list of procedures. A much
  stronger answer is to emphasise training patterns and plans,
  and to show your willingness to learn.

Procedures and ability

This is an unfortunate question as there isn't really any way of
presenting the answer other than as a list. However, this is a good
way of showing you understand the needs of the job you are
going for. Good answers tailor the list to the requirements of the
job.

- List only procedures relevant to the job for which you are
  applying.
- Absolute numbers are not necessary.
- Avoid obvious ancient history procedures such as
  catheterisation.
- Don't forget subtle things such as breaking bad news and
  dealing with difficult patient-based problems that might be
  relevant to the job you are applying for.

Duties

This word is the biggest single trap on any application form.
Universally interpreted as being simply a job description, this
question tends to produce waffly irrelevant answers that damage
the rest of the application. 'Duties' might mean absolutely
anything from turning up on time everyday, to seeing 12 patients
per outpatient clinic, to respecting duty of confidentiality to

patients. Every time I see this word on forms my heart sinks: if you have the chance to remove one question as an application form designer please remove this one. I'd be eternally grateful.

 The word 'duties' makes you think of your job description. If the shortlisters want a job description they would ask your current personnel department for one. Think before you answer this question to avoid stating the blindingly obvious.

- The only way to deal with this question is to recognise how daft it is and answer it however you like.
- Think of other criteria such as patient focus, teamworking, multiprofessional activities, etc. and sell those.
- Do not write your hours, shift pattern, on calls or daily routine.

TEACHING

Lots of different questions are posed about teaching but they are considered together. Everybody in medicine has to teach at some point. Think how you can show you are good at it, or at least enjoy it.

- Don't assume the reader understands who you are teaching.
- Indicate any teaching training or qualifications – even just a 'teaching the teachers'-type course.
- If possible, make it clear you understand the good principles of adult learning and teaching, such as gaining group buy-in for what you are covering, preparation in advance and objective setting.
- Use PPVs to identify the active role you played in coordinating and setting up teaching slots as appropriate.

MANAGEMENT

Question	Percentage of forms that asked question
1. Teamwork experience (multi-disciplinary team)	9
2. Leadership experience	8
3. Communication skills	8

Teamwork experience

Only weak CVs will not contain references to multiprofessional working and teamwork. It is an obvious place from which to sell achievements. The most effective sale here is around what you did personally to mould or develop the team, or work to solve its problems. In other words, you didn't go to a multiprofessional meeting because you were told to but because you wanted to influence it.

- Think as broadly as you can about instances where you have worked with teams.
- Remember teams that involve patients.
- Examples from outside the NHS can be used.

Leadership experience

Leadership is a difficult word to define precisely and can therefore be interpreted broadly. The more senior the job, the more detailed and wide-reaching the examples given should be. Again, consider ways in which you might be able to bring in non-NHS roles where you have demonstrated leadership.

Think of leadership as being divided into categories:

- Peer leadership: groups of students or doctors of the same peer group.

- Team or group leadership: within teams or groups of different specialist interest, motivation or discipline.
- Organisational leadership: where the whole organisation can demonstrate the influence of your leadership.
- Strategic leadership: where future outcomes and direction of teams or organisations are influenced by your leadership.

Communication skills

Communication can be divided into:

- communication with patients
- communication within teams and between healthcare professionals.

If possible, think of examples from both of these groups.

PERSONAL CRITERIA

Question	Percentage of forms that asked question
1. Provide a personal statement in support of your application	51
2. The JFK question: 'Why do you want the job?'	37
3. Can you drive?	28
4. When are you leaving your current job?	26
5. What is your current salary?	25
6. Describe any time off you have had for illness	24
7. When are you available to start in the post?	18

Personal statement

This is the most commonly asked question overall. Career plans have been included in this section.

The most important point in responding to such a question is that it doesn't read as being completely obvious or obsequious. In other words, for a putative SpR cardiology post, do not write:

> 'I seek a Calman number in cardiology with a view to becoming a consultant cardiologist.'

Nor:

> 'I seek the opportunity to train with the world-eminent Professor Smith for the best possible understanding of cardiology.'

Career plans should be succinct, relevant and interesting: and neither of the above.

Personal statements are complicated because they offer an incredibly broad opportunity, which is frequently wasted on waffle. But don't forget that you do not have to use all the space and that to leave spaces on the page is better than boring the reader to death.

Sell your big hitters again to make your portfolio interesting. If you haven't been able to include a big hitter elsewhere it will always be relevant here.

The JFK question: 'Why do you want the job?'

President John F. Kennedy, upon his inauguration, suggested to the American people that they ask not what the country can do for them but what they can do for the country.

The question 'Why do you want the job?' is one of the most frequently asked questions at interview. The best way to answer it is by answering the opposite question, 'What can I give to the job?'

You will always be asked the JFK question at least once, either in the application form or at interview and you must come up with a good answer. It is so much more powerful to hear a candidate describing what he or she can offer than to sit and listen to a long list of demands.

Can you drive?

- If your driving licence is from abroad, identify your legal right to drive in the UK.
- Unless you are asked about points on the licence or driving convictions, you do not have to list them.

When are you leaving your current job?

Although on the surface straightforward, there are some circumstances when the answer to this might not be something you want to reveal up front. For example, you might be thinking of leaving a rotation early to move up the ladder. But if you aren't successful you will continue to the end of the rotation.

What is your current salary?

We were very surprised at the number of forms that asked this question. Pay scales in the NHS are consistent between Trusts and therefore pay itself is not usually a reason for moving post. The reason for the question might be to ascertain your degree of overtime-banded pay. It seems unlikely that the answer will influence whether you are offered the post or not. Always be honest.

Describe any time off you had for illness

As with the CV, gaps on application forms are dangerous for the applicant. Unless you explain the gap, the reader will assume the worst (maybe you were in prison). So explain gaps, for family or travel reasons or anything else. And don't mix employment breaks with sickness leave – they are quite different. Prospective employers aren't going to worry about a couple of days off a year for flu but might be concerned if you took 6 months sick leave last year. Interestingly, the NHS in Wales has the highest rate of sick leave among any employer in the UK.

Summary of CVs and application forms   **10**

In this chapter

- How do you most effectively sell your achievements through the CV?
- How do you know that your CV is finished?
- How do you maximise your chances of shortlisting once the application has been delivered?

REVIEW

There are no rules on how to complete a CV, no templates to follow and no perfect CVs to copy. The objective is to keep the readers interested in your CV for as long as possible. The longer they look at the CV, the more they are likely to choose to see you rather than reject you.

The CV should be crafted with the specific job in mind, not produced 'off the shelf'. The needs of every employer are different. You wouldn't be very impressed if you went into an electrical store looking for a television and the salesman tried to sell you a dishwasher. With the CV you must ensure you are giving the information that the buyers are looking for.

WHEN IS IT FINISHED?

When you have finished writing the CV, stick it to a wall and stand a couple of metres away. What does it look like from a distance? What you are trying to work out is that the balance between writing and space is about right. CVs often have too much space

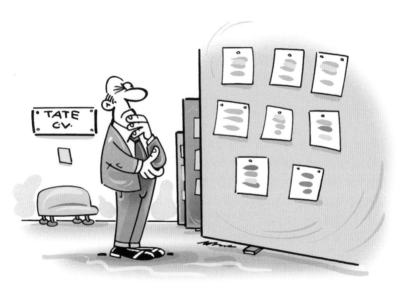

Making an impression

on the front page, making them seem short of content. On the other hand, they might be too crowded, making your mind seem cluttered. Both lead to rejection.

Do the big hitters stand out: have you put them to the left and high on the page if at all possible. And finally, is your name big enough to be clearly read at that distance?

FINAL CHECKS

- Have you removed all the sentences and put the content into bullets?
- Are all the bullets followed by positive power verbs?
- Are all the dates on the right hand side of the page?
- Have you used bold text judiciously to bring out points you want to be read?
- Have you explained anything that the recruiter won't understand – like certain prizes and awards?
- Have you thought about the outcome of your achievement and included it?
- Make sure you can explain and describe every single item listed – you might have to at interview.

GETTING OPINIONS

Everyone asks colleagues, managers, consultants or friends to review their CV. Getting opinions is useful to a point but there is the risk of getting 5 reviews and 50 opinions. And you don't want to have to change the entire CV round the night before the deadline.

 Top Tip

If getting opinions on your CV, make it clear what you want comments on. For instance, if you are sure about the layout, ask for comments on the way you have described your achievements.

At some point you have to decide the CV is finished.

Ask the expert

If I have asked one of my references to review the CV and they suggest lots of changes, is it rude if I ignore this advice?

No-one has any right to demand that your CV is presented in any specific way. There are no rules and it is your decision how to set it out. If the advice you have been given isn't helpful and you aren't going to follow it, just thank the reference for the comments without committing yourself further.

BEFORE PUTTING THE APPLICATION INTO THE POST

Check that your references know you are applying because they might be contacted at any stage and it's not helpful if they tell the recruiter they didn't know you were applying. They are supposed to be on your side after all.

Contact your references and let them know immediately that their recommendation might be called for. Send them your CV with a covering letter stating what you want them to say, remembering once again the needs of the buyers.

COVERING LETTER

You will always want to introduce your application but in general the covering letter in the medical recruitment process is nothing like as important as for jobs elsewhere. It is unlikely that your letter will be copied and sent to the panel. So don't waste time on a detailed letter: the chances of it making any difference whatsoever are miniscule.

INCREASING YOUR CHANCES AFTER YOUR APPLICATION HAS BEEN RECEIVED

This sounds impossible but it isn't. Just imagine you are in the HR department and it's closing day for a job. Your desk is covered with applications and you have perhaps a day or two to sort them and get them round to the panellists. What do you notice as you sort through all these forms?

When we collected application packs for hundreds of jobs researching this book, we were in a similar situation. Envelopes of different colours and shapes. Forms prepared well or sloppily. A neatly typed covering letter or a compliment slip. Packs put together with consideration and those thrown together willy nilly. What happened to us? We began to compare not just the content but the look of the packs, giving Papworth the highest score for presentation (see the table at the end of Chapter 6). You wanted to look at it, to find out more. The same principle applies for your application.

Top Tip
You want your application to look the best from the minute it arrives at the HR department. If you produce a really impressive looking form it will be treated preferentially. It's just human nature.

HOW TO MAKE YOUR PACK LOOK THE BEST

The best envelope

Send your application in an envelope with a stiff cardboard back. Even if the postman has squashed up everyone else's flimsy envelopes, your application will be pristine when it is reviewed. Crumpled, folded and otherwise imperfect CVs will have to fight harder against yours.

The best paper

Print the form out on good quality paper. Don't use paper that has watermarks, which risks branding the CV as owned by the company whose watermark underlies it. Choose thick paper that won't smudge if you need to write on it.

Every copy the best

Make sure that each copy of the application form and CV is copied onto the best paper. They have asked for 12 copies because it is going to 12 people and you want them all to have the pleasure of your superior presentation. Neatly clip the 12 copies together so they can be easily sorted. And if it is 12 CVs and 12 application forms use a paper clip to link the two: making it less likely that one half will get lost.

Top Tip
Place the CV on top of the application form if both are required. It is a better sell for you and brands your name (rather than the name of the Trust) from the outset.

All of these little points make your application radiate confidence and almost compel the reader to pay attention to what you are saying.

If there is any chance your pack will be late, send it by Special Delivery (which guarantees delivery before noon the day after posting) or hand-deliver it. The closing date is final and no exceptions will be made.

CONTACTING THE RECRUITER

There are reasons why you might want to contact the recruiter at this stage. Find out the name of the person in HR who is dealing with the job, call that person by his or her name, and only talk to them.

Summary

- Make sure your CV is selling your achievements for the specific job you are applying for

- Remember that opinions will be hugely varied: at some point you have to decide the CV is complete and send it off

- Make sure that your presentation looks great when it is received

The interview 11

In this chapter

- Why are interviews used to select for jobs?
- How is technique learned?
- What are the common myths about medical interviews that are false?

The interview is the Western world's method of selection. Despite constant criticism for being biased, the interview has survived. In medicine it is usually the only part of the post-shortlist stage of recruiting. Other assessment methodologies have been introduced widely in the UK (see Chapter 22) but the interview remains king.

Interviews are used because it is assumed that everyone can interview. For the recruiters they are cheap and easy to organise. Any number of people can be involved with the interview: from two consultants to a mixed-group panel of 15.

In practice, candidates for jobs are very similarly qualified. Interviewers are faced with the task of picking from a shortlist with very little to distinguish between them. Choosing between the individual candidates can be immensely difficult.

To make things worse for the interviewers, they are expected to make a decision in one sitting. They cannot recall candidates for a second stage. It is standard practice for the panel to make its selection at the end of the interview session and announce it immediately afterwards.

To be successful, you have to be better than the rest of the field. You won't get the job by being equal. And if your paper qualifications are roughly equal to those of everyone else, the only way you can perform better is by developing a winning interview technique.

> **Top tip**
> You have a much better chance of getting the job now you have been shortlisted than when you applied for the post. The odds have improved from perhaps 2 in 300 to 2 in 8. You are not starting from a weak position: always remember that the panel was interested enough in you to want to see you. Be confident in your chances.

Interviewers in medicine are almost exclusively untrained in how to interview. That offers the well-prepared candidate a really good opportunity. The questions asked are remarkably predictable. And preparation before the day of the interview is neither difficult nor time consuming.

STAGES OF EXECUTION OF THE WINNING INTERVIEW

Preparation

- Compiling lists of potential questions, categorising them and thinking about good answer strategies.

Information gathering

- Finding out as much as you can about the job, the Trust, the format of the interview, the panel and what previously successful candidates did to get the job.

Delivery, including controlling nerves

- Working out what buyers are looking for and answering questions confidently, selling your achievements effectively.

Completion and follow through

- Ending the interview well and, if unsuccessful, preparing for the next opportunity.

Each of these is described in detail over the following eight chapters.

MAKING TIME

You won't get any job without preparing for the interview. Interviews are different from examinations. You might just scrape through an exam on little or no work, but don't forget that here you cannot just pass an interview to succeed: you have to get an A.

Some of the work might have to be done during the working day. You will need to contact the hospital, make arrangements to visit, talk to the current post-holder, etc. But the rest can be done in a spare Saturday morning. You need some quiet time when you can think.

The two things you need most when thinking about preparation for the interview are:

- job description and set of evaluation criteria, if provided
- your CV.

The first gives you an indication of the broad groupings of questions you are likely to be asked. The second forms the basis for the whole of one group of questions and you must be able to explain and describe everything you have mentioned.

INTERVIEW QUESTIONS

These can be classified into three groups:

1. open/retrospective
2. aggressive/closed
3. topical.

The three styles are distinct, easy to spot and require completely different strategies in answering. A combination of different styles will be used during the interview.

COMMON MYTHS ABOUT INTERVIEWS – ALL ARE FALSE

A number of myths abound. All of the following statements about interviews in medicine *are false*:

- An internal candidate always gets the job if the decision is close.
- The bigger the panel, the more difficult the interview.
- The questions are harder if lay people are involved.
- The longer the interview, the worse it is going.
- If my reference is best mates with one of the panel I'll get the job.
- If my reference hasn't called the panel in advance I won't get the job.
- The decision is based on who has the best references.
- Ultimately, it's the quality of the CV and paper qualifications that count most.
- The most experienced candidate is most likely to be successful.
- Most medical jobs are 'sewn up' before the interviews even happen.
- Someone who is not on the panel has told the panel who they should appoint.
- You are safer with an all-medic panel.
- If the previous candidate is in the room for much longer than expected, he or she has got the job.
- You are best off if you are the first candidate to be interviewed.
- You are best off if you are the last candidate to be interviewed.

It is a complete waste of your time to worry about any of these myths. Your time is best spent preparing the way for the interview, anticipating and analysing the different questions you will be asked and polishing your technique.

Summary

- Interviews are usually the only form of post-shortlist assessment used in medical recruitment

- Interview technique is a combination of preparation, question analysis and confident delivery

Preparation for the interview

By Manoj Ramachandran

In this chapter

- Once shortlisted, how do you start preparing for the interview?
- The weeks before the interview – what should you do in advance?
- The day of the interview – what should you bring, how should you behave and what should you wear?

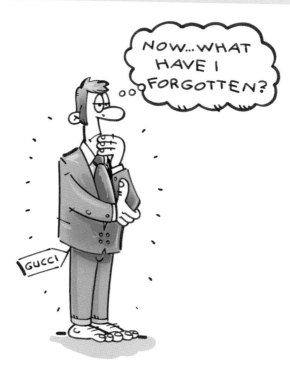

'Now, what have I forgotten?'

Your CV or application form might get you shortlisted but to get the job that you want, you must interview well on the day. Many people sell themselves well on their CV, fulfilling all the essential and most of the desired criteria on paper. But when the interview arrives they are either badly prepared or let themselves down in the stressful face-to-face situation.

Ask the expert
How do I prevent my perfect CV not resulting in getting the job?
Research and prepare for the interview in advance, and practise, practise, practise being interviewed!

PREPARING FOR THE INTERVIEW ONCE SHORTLISTED

No football manager would send a team to the World Cup final without a strategy. You must get into the mindset of planning your overall game-plan for job seeking. If you apply for more than one job and have a strong, selling CV and application form, the chances are you will be shortlisted more than once. This obviously increases your chances of getting a job, but it can also put you in the position of interviewing for a job that you might not even want. So you need to consider how to handle this situation, and whether you are going to take the job if offered it.

One solution might be to stagger jobs, so you could be offered a stand-alone A&E post but are free to attend interviews for two-to three-year rotations on the basis that you will only be starting the rotation six months later. This could allow you to avoid repeating a post such as A&E during your rotation. This strategy is particularly useful for those planning to travel for a period of time – it is better to have a job or rotation to come back to than to attend interviews while you are away.

THE INTERVIEW FORMAT

You must find out what the interview involves. You can do this by talking to the Medical Personnel officer named in the job advert, quizzing previous candidates and teasing-out information from the medical secretary of one of the interviewers. The objective is not to find out what questions are going to come up (you will be very fortunate to find that information out!) but to understand the format and set-up of the interview.

Make a list of questions to ask before you pick up the phone:

- When and where will the interview be held?
- How long will the interview be? You need to be aware of how much time you have to sell yourself.
- How many interviews are there? There is usually only one panel but in some situations, e.g. SpR interviews, there might be two or more. If you let yourself down in one of the interviews, the other panel or panels will assess you independently.
- What is the style of interview? Most interviews are simple face-to-face question-and-answer sessions. There might be a small presentation for the panel on a topic that is sent to you in advance (see Chapter 18). You might also encounter OSCE-style interviews (OSCE stands for Objective Structured Clinical Examination and is described in detail in Chapter 18).
- When will you know the results? It is important to know whether the result is announced after your interview or whether you will be notified of the decision at a later date.

THE INTERVIEW PANEL

Your next task is to find out who is on the interview panel. You should be able to get these details from Medical Personnel. Specific questions to ask are:

- How many interviewers are there in total?
- Who are the interviewers? In addition to senior medical staff, the panel could include lay members of the public, managers, staff from the Deanery, members of specialist training committees related to the post and others. They will each have a specific question to ask you; they should ask the same question to all interviewees and objectively compare the answers.
- What are the backgrounds of the medical staff? With a little bit of research and endeavour, you can find out a lot about your interviewers. You can use the Medical Register to research the educational, professional and academic background of all your interviewers. This should warn you in advance of expounding your opinions on certain topics in the interview, which might be the expert field of one of your interviewers! Further information can be found on the internet, including the individual websites of the hospitals or Trusts where the interviewers are employed.

WHAT ARE YOUR ODDS?

It seems obvious but many candidates don't know how many posts are available at a particular interview or what the candidate to job ratio is. Irrespective of the ratio, you must do a great job of selling yourself on the day to get the job. You must be better than the next best candidate.

PRACTISE, PRACTISE, PRACTISE

You must make yourself aware of the common questions that are asked frequently in interviews, and then prepare and practise answers to them. It is best to do this in front of a mirror and watch all the verbal and non-verbal cues that you emit. Close to the interview, practise with your formal suit or clothes on so that you get used to exactly what it will feel like on the day.

It is useful to practise with colleagues and seniors who have been through the interview process. Ask their advice on how to answer specific questions and get honest feedback on your technique.

If you feel you need further help, you should attend courses specifically aimed at the interview process. Try and choose one that caters to the level or specialty that you are interested in. More importantly, choose a course that offers one-to-one practise and feedback – you will find this invaluable.

If you are unlucky enough to be unsuccessful at interviews on several occasions, there is in all likelihood a problem with your interviewing technique. You are obviously good enough to be shortlisted (your CV and application form are sufficient) but you tend to let yourself down at the interview stage. Honest self-analysis is the key to success and you are most likely to benefit from individual coaching, either at a course or from an interview or life skills coach. Look out for adverts for such services in trade magazines like *BMJ Careers, Hospital Doctor* and *GP*.

PREPARING ON THE DAY OF THE INTERVIEW

Come the big day, there are several points to consider before you even step into the interview room.

What should you bring?

The following is a list of items that you should consider bringing with you to your interview:

- The letter confirming your interview – know exactly where the interviews are being held, and take a map of the location if you haven't been there before.
- A copy of your CV – you are often asked to bring this along but it is helpful to refresh your memory. Make a list of the big hitters you want to sell and bring this list along too.

- Documents requested by the interview panel – including copies of your certificates, course attendance confirmations and publications. A leather-bound portfolio with loose leaves into which you can insert the requested documents ensures that the documents are easy to handle and adds a professional sheen to how you are perceived.
- Passport photographs – these are often requested by Medical Personnel. Get these well in advance to avoid a mad search for photo booths on the day!

Getting there

I cannot adequately emphasise the importance of knowing exactly where the interview venue is. If possible, you should aim to get there at least 45 minutes in advance. Any earlier and you might have to suffer the stress of a prolonged and nervous wait with your fellow interviewees. Any later and you might be cutting it too fine. Remember that the interviews can often run early or late and you might be called for at a time that you do not expect – so arrive in good time.

If you have never been to the venue before it might be possible to do a dry run before the interview. Listen out for travel updates before you set off on the day itself. If all this sounds obvious, let me assure you that I have met several candidates who have either missed an interview altogether (usually because they had to travel a great distance) or have turned up late. Being late might be excused if you have a good enough reason but it certainly does not set a good precedent for the kind of employee that you are going to be.

YOU ARE YOU BEING WATCHED...

The interview starts the moment you appear within the surroundings of the venue. As far as you are concerned, you are being watched at all times. People who are part of the interview process (e.g. Medical Personnel and members of the interview panel) might be travelling to the venue at the same time as you. If you behave in a manner that is unbecoming (e.g. being rude to fellow passengers on the train) this will be noted.

When you enter the venue itself, receptionists and Medical Personnel/Staffing officers might also be watching your every move. The latter have direct contact with the interview panel, so watch how you behave in front of them.

You must behave appropriately around the other candidates too. For a nervous candidate, there is nothing more infuriating than a bunch of 'mates' openly discussing the interview, assessing their chances and loudly discussing their lives in the waiting area. Equally, there are those who insist on assessing their competitors' chances by direct questioning. This can again be very annoying. It is safer to be quiet and discreet. Only speak when you are spoken to and speak as little as possible.

DON'T FORGET...

You know your body and you know how it behaves in stressful situations. So be aware of:

- Perspiration – some people sweat a lot in stressful situations, while others don't. Learn how to control sweat as far as you can. Make sure that at least your hands are free of sweat when you go in to shake the interviewers' hands. Go to the bathroom and wash and dry your hands immediately before the interview.
- Ablutions – suffice it to say that you shouldn't need to ask for the restroom in the middle of the interview.
- Posture and presence – make sure you stand up straight when you walk into the interview room. Poise is a difficult characteristic to teach but it is something you must be aware of.

- Smile –smile often and appropriately! Do not smile inanely at the interviewers just because you feel the need to smile constantly.
- Don't forget to switch pagers, bleeps, mobile phones and any other electronic or communication devices off before you walk in.

WHAT YOU SEE IS WHAT YOU GET (WYSIWYG)

Think hard about how you will appear and what you will be wearing to the interview. Stand in front of a mirror and look at yourself from top to bottom:

- Hair – for men, make sure your hair is kept neat and trimmed. For women, as a general rule, control of your hair is more important than the exact style, appearance or length. Try not to fiddle with your hair during the interview – this might be interpreted as a sign of nervousness.
- Personal hygiene – make sure you have thought about the length of your fingernails, dandruff, body odour and breath. Try not to flood the interview room with your favourite perfume or aftershave.
- Handshake – use a firm handshake (not too soft or hard) and, importantly, shake hands with the interviewers only if they offer their hands to you. It can be interpreted as quite aggressive to enter the room and offer your hand immediately to all the interviewers.

The following are general rules only. Ultimately, it is your decision what to wear – go with what makes you feel confident on the day.

For men

- Suit – buy (if you don't have one already) a well-fitted suit and make sure it looks neat and pressed on the day.

Choose a dark suit (black, charcoal grey or dark blue) to appear as neutral as possible.

- Shirt – try to wear a white or light blue shirt as neutral colours. Avoid white shirts with a black suit – you may look as if you are going to your own funeral! It does not matter whether you wear cufflinks. If you choose to, avoid anything that might be considered offensive (I once saw a candidate wearing a pair of cufflinks with the words 'arse' and 'elbow' on them in an interview – not the wisest of choices!).
- Tie – again, choose something neutral and inoffensive. Avoid ties with logos, garish designs and club emblems (e.g. rugby, cricket, hockey and football team ties) – you might offend as many people as you think you are attracting. Avoid bow ties.
- Shoes and socks – shine your shoes and wear dark socks if possible.
- Accessories and jewellery – men should keep accessories and jewellery to an absolute minimum.
- Make-up –best avoided in men.

For women

- Suit – it does not matter whether you wear a trouser suit or one with a skirt. Generally, avoid very short skirts. Be aware of where your skirt is when crossing and uncrossing your legs. The exact colour of your suit does not matter as long as it appears smart.
- Blouses – again, the exact colour does not matter as long as it is coordinated with your suit.
- Neckwear/scarves – as discretion is the order of the day, avoid flamboyant neckwear.
- Shoes –the same rules apply as above.
- Stockings/tights – bring a spare pair just in case of last-minute laddering, or wear a trouser suit

- Accessories and jewellery – coordinate with your suit and avoid going over the top.
- Make-up – this is up to the individual candidate and is very difficult to advise on!

Summary

- You need to prepare well in advance of your interview

- Tasks you should consider include finding out in advance about the format of the interview, the interview panel and preparing an overall strategy in your approach to the jobseeking process

- Make sure you think carefully about what items to bring with you to the interview, how to behave when you get there and what to wear on the day

13

How do they decide?

In this chapter

- What factors influence the decision makers on the other side of the interview table?
- How do you handle a situation in which there seems to be a favoured internal candidate?
- What are the basic theories behind selection by interview?

HOW DO YOU GET A JOB?

Although you should assume when going through the interview that this alone generates success, the panel still has access to your application form, which might be referred back to, especially if the decision is tight. Your big hitters, carefully deployed in the application form, might still win the day.

There are three circumstances you might encounter at interview:

1. The panel has already made up its mind who to appoint: the interview is just for show.
2. There are a number of stronger candidates amongst the shortlisted group, from which subset the panel expects to appoint.
3. The panel is considering every applicant equally and enters the process with no preconceived ideas who to appoint.

The first circumstance is considered later in the chapter. You must treat the second two circumstances equally: even if there is a subset of stronger candidates, you have no way of knowing whether you are in it or not. It is fruitless to speculate and a waste of time to prepare for the interview in any other way than by polishing your technique.

WHAT IS THE PANEL LOOKING FOR?

Examining what the panel is likely to expect from the successful candidate is an art, but there are several clues which you can find with minimal research.

1. Information packs

When the job application form was posted to you an information pack was probably enclosed. This might include a list of essential and desirable criteria. These criteria have been decided upon by the employing Trust and agreed by the panel. It is unlikely you would even have been shortlisted without all the essential criteria. However, the more of the desirable list you can tick, or partially tick as 'work in progress,' the higher your chance.

2. Current post-holder

What kind of person does this panel have a track record of recruiting? How did the current post-holder get the job? If the interview panel is same as six or twelve months ago, what kind of questions were asked?

3. Job success maps

It is useful to map the requirements that the panel will have for the job: part of this will come from the information pack. Try to think laterally about what the requirements might be that perhaps have not been considered openly. Think of the possibilities under headings:

Clinical experience	Remember, this is usually the least discriminating factor
Decision making	If you will be responsible for delivery of services
Team working	Will the rest of the team get on well with you?
Academic background	Do you have a track record of instigating serious research which builds a unit's reputation?
Management ability	Can you successfully take on management responsibility?
Clinical governance	A big burden of work for all departments which you would be well placed to contribute to
Communication and patient-focused activities	Something others may not have considered

Once you have mapped the likely needs of the job, try to plug your own big hitters into the framework you have created. In how many of these (and other) boxes can you offer something?

WHAT IF THEY HAVE ALREADY MADE UP THEIR MINDS?

Often you get a feeling that the panel has already made up its mind who to appoint. Candidates who might have been pre-selected for success include:

- a well known internal candidate
- someone coming with a reputation
- an individual who was passed over at the previous interview but 'promised' the job the next time round

- a candidate who has a world class, unbeatable application form and CV
- an individual who fits the profile for the vacancy exactly: perhaps because of complementary areas of a speciality (particularly in consultant interviews).

HOW CAN YOU TELL IF THE PANEL ISN'T REALLY GIVING YOU A LOOK-IN?

There is absolutely nothing you can do about it if the interview process is fixed from the start. You should never assume anything though, and it is possible that if you perform well you will be successful despite a precluded panel view. If you perform much better than all the other candidates you should get the job.

Top Tip

Never assume you have been unsuccessful. Always perform to your highest ability in the interview. Even if someone has been pre-selected, you might get the job by performing better than everyone else on the day. And even if your fears are correct, all interview experience is positive in that it helps you rehearse for the next time, when your chances will be higher

Clues implying the decision has already been made include:

- Interviewers talking to each other as you answer, or even getting up and leaving.
- Constant interruptions during the interview.
- Closed, loaded comments like 'You aren't as experienced as the other candidates we are seeing today'.
- Suggestions on other jobs to consider applying for, before returning to interview for this post again in six or twelve months.

INTERNAL CANDIDATES

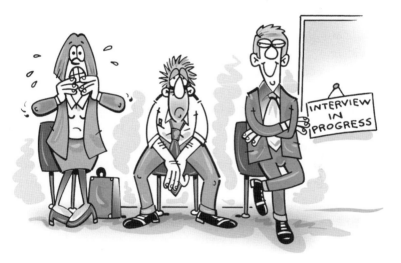

'Who's the internal candidate?'

A particular worry of many applicants is the presence of a favoured internal candidate, usually someone who is currently employed at a lower grade and who is poised for promotion. You might have been told by one of the current incumbents for the position that you have 'no chance' of success because the consultants have already indicated they want someone whom they know. There is the old maxim, 'better the devil you know' which many applicants assume is always the default position of interview panels.

What the current post-holder says is informative but comes without any teeth. He or she might have badly misinterpreted the status of your competitor. Perhaps this individual has gone round the mess telling everyone he or she is a 'shoe-in' for the job and your informer has believed this. If the employing consultants have also heard this rumour it is likely to act against the internal candidate.

It is probably true that internal candidates have a starting advantage. It's exactly the same as a home football game or a British player competing at Wimbledon. In some ways this is entirely natural, and it works for you, too, if you decide to apply for a further job in the same hospital as you currently work.

But interviews are conducted in a way that tends to narrow the opening advantage the internal candidate has. Some are so structured that all candidates are asked exactly the same questions and so good technique wins. You might find, when you actually attend the interview, that it seems to be a foregone conclusion – as above. However, you might be pleasantly surprised that the process is completely transparent.

Don't get put off by the internal candidate. His or her advantage is at best minimal and can usually be trumped by really good interview technique.

INTERVIEW SELECTION THEORY

Academic human resources units have concluded that there are two patterns of decision-making amongst interviewers.

Sometimes, different members of any interview panel divide into both categories, in which case the chair might decide which pattern is dominant:

1. 30-second window – a decision is made in the first 30 seconds of the interview whether a candidate is going to be successful or not. Often, the rest of the interview is rather unstructured, as if clutching at straws to find some questions with which to fill the time.
2. Gradual summation – this is an additive interview where answers are listened to and used to build an overall picture. The panel might ask everyone similar questions. Although perceived as fairer, this also tends to flatten the field somewhat, making it more difficult to demonstrate a really strong performance.

Attribute	30-second window interviews	Gradual summation interviews
Start of interview	Confident start vital	Confident start less vital
Way you sit, posture and attitude	More likely to be beneficial (not much else to go on)	Less important: serves to make you feel more confident rather than in deciding the outcome
First question	Direct and slightly unusual: only the answers at the very beginning count	Probably open: designed to relax you and get you talking
Structure	Less clear: sometimes seems random	Clearer, planned, definite
Length	Often shorter and may finish abruptly	Fixed: and roughly the same for each candidate

SELECTION PANELS

There are three patterns:

1. two consultants interviewing together
2. more than two consultants in a panel form
3. panel format with interviewers from different backgrounds (e.g. hospital management, lay people).

Two consultants format

- Frequently used at entry-level interviews, for PRHO and SHO jobs.
- Likely to be consultants with whom the interviewee will eventually work.
- Formality, time-keeping and efficiency of organisation highly variable and can run over time.
- Tends to favour internal or very strong candidates.

Multiple consultants panel

- This often implies a political imperative that groups of consultants all have a say in an appointment.
- Used extensively for SHO rotations where consultants come from different hospitals.
- Very unlikely that any given candidate will be known by all.
- One or two dominant figures can have a great deal of sway over the others.

Multiprofessional panel

- Almost always used for consultant and SpR level interviews.
- Hospital chief executive or representative is present.
- Lay people often present too – it is important that you do not use medical jargon as it might be interpreted as an inability to communicate.

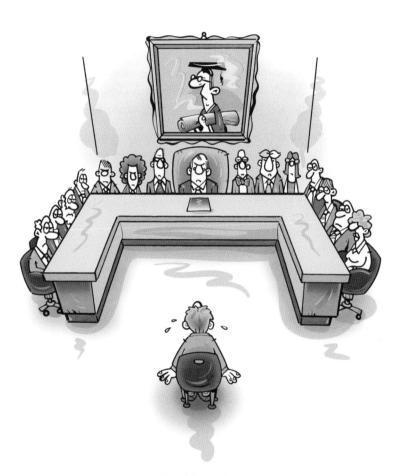

Panel interviews

- Much more structured: often with questions distributed equally around the group.
- Acts extensively against internal candidates.

Summary

- It is possible to predict the types of characteristics that a successful candidate for any given post is likely to demonstrate and there are ways of researching these

- Do not assume that an internal candidate has an advantage – but be able to recognise when the decision to appoint someone else has already been taken

- Understand the different styles of interview and types of group that candidates should expect

5 minutes before and 1 minute after

14

In this chapter

- What techniques can you use to avoid getting flustered immediately before an interview?
- How will the interview begin?
- How do you get out of an interview safely?

STRESS BUILDING UP

Stress actually starts to build subconsciously the day the brown envelope arrives with a date for the interview. Despite being pleased to be shortlisted, you also begin to get nervous.

Nerves build further the night before – as you get your clothes ready – and even further through the day the interview is to be held. But you experience greatest anxiety as you see the preceding candidate return from interview and you are asked by the administrator to get ready.

5 MINUTES TO GO

You might have brought material to look through while you wait. The most useful preparation tool is a few small cards on which you list your big hitters and what you plan to say about them. In the last 5 minutes, review the list you have written. Think about the times when these big hitters occurred – how you felt and what the achievement meant to you. Think positively about how you would like to describe these achievements.

Interview technique can be taught – just like clinical examinations. The agenda of any interview is controlled by the panel and your ability to influence this agenda is key to your chances of success.

Obviously, your best bet is to talk to your strengths. You have already decided (at the time of writing your CV) what your big hitters are. The same big hitters apply to the interview. The more of these you can get into the discussion, the longer you can talk about them and the more interested the panel are in hearing about them, the better for you. So introducing a big hitter at any point in the interview is really good technique.

Top Tip
The last place you should visit before going into the interview room is the bathroom. Wash you hands and dry them thoroughly. You might be asked to shake hands and (believe me) there is absolutely nothing worse for a member of an interview panel to shake a sweaty, dripping appendage. A good handshake is a great start.

DELAYS AND HOLD-UPS

It is very common for you to be held up outside the interview room for a few minutes. It is easy at this point to conclude:

- That they are spending ages talking about the preceding candidate (i.e. that person has got the job and you haven't).
- That they are looking through your information and planning lots of really difficult questions (i.e. they don't want you to get the job).

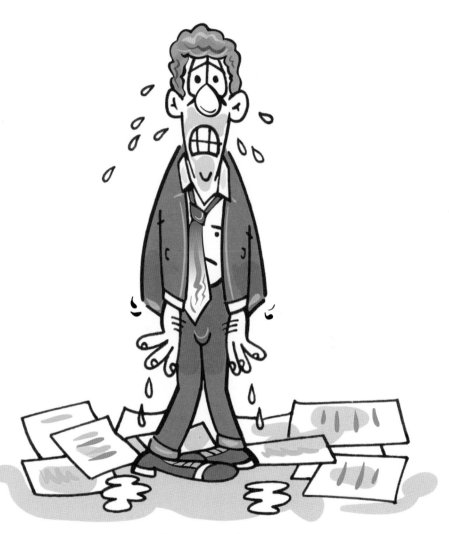

It'll be a piece of cake

It is, in fact, much more likely that one of the panel has gone to the bathroom, or to check the tennis scores, or that a cup of coffee is being served. Don't get flustered if there is a delay. Read your cards of big hitters again and focus on the positives.

WALKING THROUGH THE DOOR

The door might be held open or you might have to open it yourself. Watch what happened when other candidates were escorted into the interview. Just like the story about working out how to adjust the couches for clinical exams so you don't look stupid in front of an examiner, work out how to open and close the door without attracting attention. Thank the administrator if he or she takes you into the room.

SHAKING HANDS

Remember that you have entered the panel's room; it is in the panel's gift to award the job and you want to behave in a way that is concordant with the tone it has set. If panel members want to shake hands with you they will offer their hand, but don't force yourself on people – it is embarrassing for everyone.

SITTING DOWN

I always get a laugh when I tell people I am going to show them how to sit. But looking confident while seated in an uncomfortable chair in the middle of a hostile room is difficult. In advance of the interview, practise sitting in a hard chair and looking at your posture in the mirror. Be careful with your hands – and don't contort your body by crossing legs and leaning forward. That just looks nervous. Try to adopt a posture that is confident and professional but not aggressive.

Most importantly don't sit down until you are asked to. Often, there are several empty chairs in the room. Some might belong to absent members of the panel, others might have been used earlier for a seminar and not stacked. The chair of the panel will know where you need to sit. Even if there is only one chair, wait to the side of it until you are asked to sit. After all, you wouldn't walk into the house of your boyfriend's or girlfriend's parents for the first time, march into their sitting room and sit down before being invited to. This is the panel's room and the panel's rules. Don't risk being asked to stand up again or sitting in the wrong chair – it just gets things off to a dreadful start.

 Your hands give you away. Every other part of your body might be calm and collected but if you are nervous your hands will shake and you will wring them. When seated, keep your hands apart. And never take a glass of water – it's the most obvious trap in the book because the members of the panel can see clearly how nervous you are. If they are really lucky your hands will shake so much you'll drop the water all over yourself. No beverages.

THE LAST MINUTE OF THE INTERVIEW

The same principles apply to the conclusion as to the start. Wait to be asked to leave before getting up, shake hands again only if hands are proffered. Thank the panel members for their time. And don't look back when you have left the table. After all, you don't want to see them shaking their heads or (worse) laughing at your performance.

It is really important that you know before the interview whether the panel is expecting you to stay behind so that they can announce the successful candidates. Personally, I think this is horrific. It reminds me of the day I passed the MRCS. Successful

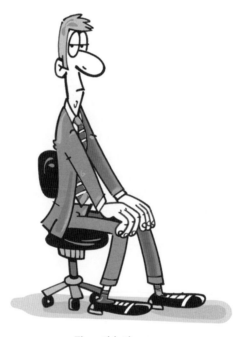

The athletic pose

candidates were called and asked to go into another room (where there was sherry) and those who had not passed were left outside like the people on a packed platform of the tube at rush hour who can't get into the crowded cars and have to wait for the next one.

But you need to know, partly for logistical reasons (trains home, etc.) and also because it dictates what happens at the end of the interview. If you are going to be informed of the decision by post, leave the hospital immediately. If you are meeting friends, arrange somewhere offsite to meet. The quicker you leave the sooner you forget and move on. If you were successful, fine. Otherwise you need to be able to pick yourself up and work on the next interview.

Don't ruminate on your performance. Tomorrow's another day.

Summary

- Stay positive just before the interview begins by focusing on your big hitters

- Wait before sitting down and shake hands only if they are offered

- At the end of the interview, leave the hospital straight away unless you have to wait for the results to be announced later on

Open/retrospective questions

15

In this chapter

- What are the different styles of interview question and how are they identified?
- What are the pitfalls of the open/retrospective style of questioning?
- How can you prepare effectively for these questions?

Having got as far as sitting in the chair, the rest of the interview involves listening to, interpreting and answering a series of questions. Although the range of questions is enormous, all of them can be clustered into three groups:

1. open/retrospective questions
2. topical questions
3. aggressive/closed questions.

Each style of questioning has its merits and normally a combination of styles will be employed. Sometimes, different members of the panel will ask contrasting styles of question. Alternatively, the same interviewer will switch from one type to another, unsettling the interviewee in the process.

OPEN/RETROSPECTIVE QUESTIONS

These are by far the most commonly employed in medical interviews. Most interviews open with this style and many never switch from this style before the end.

The biggest clue that this style is being used actually comes from the waiting room (unless you are the first candidate in). Previously I advised spending as little time in the waiting room as possible, and certainly not saying much about the interview. But one thing happens without any prompting.

When candidates return to the waiting room they give their overall impression of the interview. Some might try to unnerve their competitors by exaggerating how difficult the interview had been. But most are not so calculating. Think back to how many times you have been overheard a candidate saying 'they were so nice'. This indicates they had the open/retrospective style of interview.

So this style is also known as the 'they were so nice' style.

BASIC PRINCIPLES

Focused on you

All the questions are about you and your achievements. You are occasionally asked about the activities of a team. Questions are all phrased so the interviewer can gain more information about what you did, why you did it and what you learnt from it.

Time sensitive

By definition, you can't have achievements in the future and so the questions relate to the past. Specific moments in time (or periods, like a single job or a single decision) are explored in detail. You are never expected to expand on how you would deal with an as-yet undiscovered situation.

Deals with motivation

Most of the questions explore what you did with a specific job, or opportunity, so that the interviewer can gauge your degree of commitment and motivation. This style can sometimes feel a bit like a psychiatry history.

RECOGNISING THE STYLE

All the questions begin with an open-ended stem:

- Tell me about . . .
- Tell me more about . . .
- What made you decide to . . . ?
- Why did you . . . ?
- I see that you did . . . , what was it that convinced you to do that . . . ?

All the questions are set in the past in some way: either a discrete occasion or a period.

The questions are always about you. You are never asked to speculate or predict or theorise, just to give examples from your past. Your reasoning behind decisions might be analysed but not in a hostile way.

You find yourself relaxing as you hear the first question and continuing to open up as the questions continue. Your mind tells you that 'this isn't nearly so bad as I thought' and you conclude that the panel is 'nice'.

Finally, you do most of the talking. The answer to a single question could theoretically occupy the entire interview if you continued to talk. But even if the interviewer does ask another open question the stems are usually short and you can – and should – give extensive and detailed answers. By the end of the interview you have done perhaps 90% of the talking. Often, the interviewer sits there nodding, or making notes, throughout.

COMMON PITFALLS

Although the least overtly stressful of the three styles, this is by far the hardest in which to impress – because the questions are about you and it is uncomfortable to sell yourself properly. It isn't really part of British culture, after all, to 'boast' about your past. Perhaps they will think you are arrogant.

Not selling yourself

The most common reaction to this style is, therefore, to undersell. In a competitive field, open/retrospective questioning is the least discriminating because it tends to level the group. Candidates can easily underprepare for this style of questioning, focusing instead on preparation for the other two styles of question.

 It is incredibly easy to sell something or someone else in answering this style. For instance, 'Tell me about your job at the Chelsea and Westminster Hospital' can too easily be answered by discussing how new, attractive, vibrant, cultured and well-placed for restaurants and bars the hospital is. And answering a question about a job with Professor Jones is frequently answered by describing what a world leader Professor Jones is. He can sell himself.

Focusing on the negatives

Even worse than not selling yourself is the tendency for you actually to offer negatives about your past to the panel. We don't like to 'boast' and consider that it is more sensible to be 'measured' about what we have done in the past. So it is tempting to say things like, 'I wish I had more time to . . . ,' 'I should have got involved with more research', etc.

Stating the obvious

The other problem is the tendency to answer the question with an answer that is completely obvious. For instance:

'Why do you want the job?'

Answered as:

> 'I have now completed my basic medical training and seek a post as a specialist registrar in cardiology with a view to becoming a cardiology consultant.'

Of course, there is nothing untrue about this answer but if the first part of the answer wasn't true you wouldn't have been shortlisted. And if the second part isn't true why on earth would you want a cardiology rotation?

Boring, repetitive answers

It can be difficult to think of examples to describe experiences and motivations, especially when applying for the first few jobs of a career. But constantly repeating the same details to illustrate a point is hardly inspiring for the interviewer, especially when prefaced by 'As I said a few minutes ago . . .'

COMMON QUESTIONS

Top Tip
The most common question of all in this group is the JFK question: 'Why do you want the job'. Personally, I believe this is the fairest question – after all why on earth should anyone give you a job if you don't know why you want it. If I am ever asked for help in answering one single question this is it. But remember to answer the JFK question by turning it round to 'What can I give to the job?' (see Chapter 9).

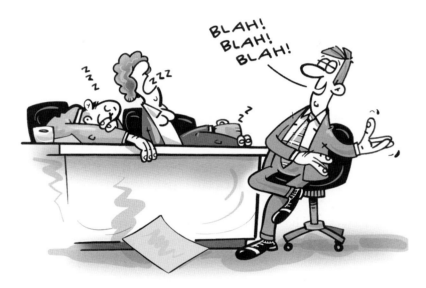

'As I said a few minutes ago . . .'

Other common questions include:

- Tell me about your current post.
- What made you decide to apply for this job?
- What made you choose the rotation/job you are doing now?
- What experience of teaching and training have you had?
- What were the highlights of your medical school life?
- What made you go into medicine?
- Looking back over your career so far, what would you consider your strengths to be?
- What are your interests outside of work?
- I see you sing in a choir, tell me more about that.
- How has your first house officer post been?
- Tell me a bit more about yourself.
- Have you been involved in any research?
- Does you unit undertake any audit work?
- What do you know about this job?

POLISHING YOUR TECHNIQUE

As soon as you hear the open/retrospective stem, train yourself to hear a warning bell. Although the question is 'nice', you must be selling effectively to be successful.

Sell yourself

It might not feel natural to sell yourself in an interview and the questions may seem innocuous, so it is easy to consider the interview as just a conversation – which it is not.

Selling yourself in the interview is exactly the same as when writing a CV:

- Work out what the buyer is in the market to buy.
- Demonstrate that you have the features they are looking for.

- Describe and augment relevant experiences.
- Don't forget that you can always discuss non-medical aspects of your past.
- Bring in and sell your list of big hitters.

 Top Tip
Remember the headhunter's maxim: past performance is the best predictor of future performance. You have to demonstrate a clear track-record of achievement and delivery in this style of interview to convince the panel members you will deliver again – this time for them.

Bring on the big hitters

In Chapter 14, I advised reviewing the list of big hitters you have prepared as the last thing you do before entering the room. This is the type of interview that they are needed for. Use the openness of the questions to get your big hitters – which play to your strengths and therefore sell you – onto the agenda. With a bit of luck, the interviewer will be 'led' by this and continue to ask you about your own big hitters for several more questions. You are much better off on this ground than somewhere else the interviewer chooses. In general, good technique is demonstrated when you have been able to bring up your big hitters and develop them.

Be imaginative

Think of the broadest, widest possible set of circumstances you could draw upon, don't just think about one strength or one achievement. The more imaginative you are with the descriptions of your motivations – what, who, why, where, when – the more impressive your answers will be.

Teach yourself to stop talking

As the answer goes on it begins to get less interesting and often in this style the interviewer does not interrupt. When you have concluded what you are going to say, stop talking. Even if there is a pregnant silence, just wait for the interviewer to ask the next question. At the very least it will force him or her to listen to the first part of your next answer.

Match the situation in the past to one in the future (in the job you are applying for)

Despite focusing on the past, the questions you will be asked are exploring your suitability for the job for which you are being interviewed. Try and think about what the challenges of the next job will be and demonstrate through your examples that you have experience in meeting similar challenges. This will reassure the panel that you are competent and trustworthy, and likely to perform.

Be interesting

Nobody wants to be bored to death and if you cannot think of anything interesting to say in a 15-minute interview you are not likely to do much better over 6 months. It is human nature to be interested in others and you should tap into this.

Inspire them

You are trying to get the panel to buy into you personally. Think of television interviews with individuals you have been inspired by. What was it that was so impressive? Perhaps it was the obvious enjoyment they got out of something, or the energy they put in. It might be the sheer determination and hard work they demonstrated. Almost definitely they came across as people you want to spend more time with. If you are awarded the job, the panel will certainly have to spend more time with you.

Summary

- Open/retrospective questions are also the 'they were so nice' questions

- Although innocuous on the surface, several traps can emerge

- Answer the questions by selling your past achievements effectively, remembering that these best predict how you will perform in the next job

Topical questions

16

- How do you recognise a topical question?
- Given the degree of interest in the NHS, how can you prepare for these questions?
- What is the best technique for answering?

The NHS is one of the biggest topics of conversation in British politics. It is an organisation about which everyone has an opinion, most think they have the answers and no-one entirely agrees. Much of the opinion expressed about the NHS reflects a political standpoint, whether liberal or conservative. As employees of the NHS, doctors are in the unusual position of both being entitled an opinion about it from the point of view of being informed members of the public and also gaining a living from it.

It isn't surprising that topical questions are moving much higher up the agenda in the interview process for medical jobs. Asking questions about the NHS, and topical events within it, allows the interviewer to gauge the respondent's intelligence, grasp of complex issues and analytical powers. In other words, this line of questioning is close to the characteristics that define the job that interviewees are applying for.

There is absolutely no doubt that these questions can be prepared for. But prepared answers are not the same as good interview technique. Many doctors prepare 'stock' answers, trying their best to predict the answer they think the interviewer wants to hear. Unfortunately, they often fall down when the questioning gets more involved and the superficiality of their understanding is laid bare.

BASIC PRINCIPLES

Topical

The questions all relate to healthcare policy, doctors' employment or remuneration, current press ruminations and alternatives to current political thought.

Different questions for different grades

The questions asked for different grades of doctor are largely the same in the other two styles but here the questions will be significantly different. The longer an individual doctor has worked in the NHS, the more of a view – and the more views – he or she will have about it. And strategy, NHS structure and policy implementation are more pertinent to more senior doctors. Although it is impossible to predict exactly what questions are asked at which grade of interview, there are some general principles:

- Topical, hospital-specific issues (impact of new building or department, utilisation of nurse consultants, link to teaching units) are more common questions for doctors in training.
- Medical workforce issues (hours, conditions, pay, multidisciplinary working) are also frequently asked of doctors in training.
- NHS-wide policy and strategy issues are more common in SpR and especially in consultant interviews.

Universal language

One big advantage to this style of questioning is that, in a mixed profession panel where managers and lay people are present, it is much easier to ensure that no jargon is used. The interview could be transposed directly to other healthcare professional groups. Members of the panel do not have to have a specific understanding of the medical profession or training to be able to participate.

Public domain

All the questions within this section reflect issues that any informed member of the public could research and form opinions about. Some are relatively profession-specific (working hours, contracts of employment, multiprofessional working). But others relate more to policy and politics (NHS funding, private health, waiting times). A well-informed medical journalist on a national paper would probably have a better grasp of the issues than the average interviewer.

Opinion

It is essential to understand that these questions are not aimed at testing your factual understanding of a topical issue *per se*. Instead, they are assuming that you have enough of a grasp of the subject to be able to discuss it intelligently and express opinion(s) about it.

RECOGNISING THE STYLE

The questions are posed in a similar way to a media interview in which your opinion and views on an issue are canvassed. This style is the easiest to recognise because it is usually transparent and the topic that is chosen for debate is normally introduced by the interviewer. One exception is if you inadvertently 'drop' an issue into the answer to one of the other two styles of question. If this happens, the interviewer might pick it up and question you further on it.

Top Tip
If you are well prepared, a topical interview will give you the best chance to shine. Use any opportunity you can to try to switch from open/retrospective or aggressive/closed styles into the topical style. Do this by dropping a topic you are comfortable talking about into the answer you give to one of the other styles of question. Hopefully (and fortunately usually) the interviewer will take the bait.

The question might openly ask for an opinion. Alternatively, it might address one specific subsection of an issue: in which case you have the option of either keeping your answer very narrow or broadening it to encompass more of the topic. The latter is a better technique if you know a lot about the subject chosen.

COMMON PITFALLS

Too rehearsed

Many interviewees make a mistake of learning answers to predicted questions parrot fashion and then reciting them like a French verb table. Although this certainly reduces the chance of clamming up and not being able to say anything at all, it is also totally obvious even to inexperienced interviewers. Good interviewers realise the answer is rehearsed and then ask the next couple of questions in a way that no-one could have predicted as a way of catching the over-rehearsed interviewee out. Rehearse the arguments but not the exact words you are going to use.

Giving them the answer you think they want to hear

With many of these questions there is no right or wrong answer. After all, they deal with opinion. But many interviewees believe they can predict what the interviewer wants to hear and then simply gives them that answer. The best example is below:

'What do you think about the reduction in junior doctors' hours?'

To which the answer given is:

'I am against it: it never hurt anyone to work hard and consultants are better trained if they worked long hours as a junior.'

In this style what is interesting to the interviewer is to hear different or lateral views and then debate them. The point is not to simply agree with everything the interviewer says but to be able to debate the answers.

Getting into a fight

Many interviewers will instinctively play 'devil's advocate' in this type of interview. Whatever opinion you give they immediately say they support the opposite. If you say you believe in private practice they immediately say they oppose it, so to assess your ability to understand an opposing view and deal with it. Sticking with your view is fine, but some interviewers can goad you into becoming angry with their opinion, especially if (deliberately) stated in an arrogant or patronising way. This is a trap: whatever happens don't let the interviewer make you angry.

Fickle opinions

This is the exact opposite of the above. When the devil's advocate opinion is given, the interviewee simply apologises and agrees with the interviewer. This gives the impression that the interviewee either doesn't have an opinion at all or doesn't want to debate it. Either way you have presented a weakness and are likely to fail.

COMMON QUESTIONS

 By definition, the potential issues for debate change rapidly. The best way to prepare is by keeping an eye on stories in the medical and national press.

- What do you think of the NHS?
- Do you think there are alternatives to the NHS for healthcare provision in the UK?
- What are your views on clinical governance?
- Many doctors think switching over to the US model for funding health would be a good idea – do you agree?
- Do you approve of the private finance initiative?
- What are the specific advantages and disadvantages of foundation status for NHS Trusts?
- Do you think elected boards of governors for hospitals are a good idea?
- How long should patients have to wait for treatment?
- Should private practice be allowed?
- What do you think of the reduction of doctors' hours that has been the result of the implementation of the European Working Time Directive?
- What will be the effects of revalidation of doctors by the GMC?
- Do you agree that nurses should progress their careers into matrons and nurse consultants, and what are the implications for junior doctor training?
- How can the culture of litigation in the NHS be stemmed?
- Do you think Foundation Programmes will improve PRHO and SHO training or not?

POLISHING TECHNIQUE

Pros and cons

Most topical questions offer two opposing possible responses, with variations. Some (like the financing of healthcare in the UK) have lots of possible solutions. Given that you recognise the question and understand the likelihood that the interviewer will listen to your opinion and then give the opposite, you can pre-empt this by putting both opinions onto the table at once.

Top Tip
Pros and cons technique
Whenever a topical question requiring an opinion is posed, pause to reflect on both sides of the argument. Then offer both contrasting opinions, with the pros stated first. This creates an early impression that you are measured enough to be able to understand the basics behind both sides of the argument.

Using the pros and cons technique is the most effective way of achieving this.

Plan the topics

As discussed above, you should never rehearse arguments. But you can reliably predict what topics are likely to come up by keeping up with the news, skimming through the medical press. If you get into the habit of doing this all the time then issues won't suddenly appear before the interview. And if you don't understand 'what all the fuss is about' with a given issue then take the time to research it.

Coffee shop, bar and home

The other really good advantage to this style of questioning is that it simulates conversation you might have with anyone, anywhere. So in preparing for the interview get your friends to argue from the opposing side from you so that you can test the depth of your understanding of the issues. They don't necessarily have to be that familiar with the issues: just be able to see what the other side of the argument is likely to be.

Having a conversation not an interview

An interview is not the same as a conversation; it is never equal. But in this particular style the best outcome is to be discussing the issue with the interviewer in a similar way as you would with friends. In other words, you are demonstrating your ability to communicate evenly with the interviewer. This is a very strong position to get into because it leaves the impression that when given the job you will be able to get on socially with the employer.

Say you don't know

It is quite possible that you will never have heard of the topic brought up. Perhaps the private finance initiative has never really reached beyond the subconscious. In this situation simply tell the interviewer you don't know what the topic is. Under no circumstances try to guess.

If you say you don't know anything about the subject, expect the interviewer to move on to another topical question. Of course, if you keep on saying that you don't know to repeated questions you will leave an impression that you are like an ostrich with your head in the sand while the daily issues of the NHS march past. Ultimately, the point of this style of questioning is to test that you do have some understanding of the environment in which you work, so hopefully there will only be one 'I don't know' during the interview.

No jargon

Be very careful and avoid trying to 'medicalise' the topical answer. It is not intended to test medical knowledge and the non-medical members of the panel will be left out and thus less likely to give you their vote at the end of the afternoon.

Summary

- Topical questions are good for the prepared candidate because they offer a unique opportunity to develop an almost equal relationship with the interviewer

- Be careful not to over-rehearse, but gain a grasp of all the issues within the medical and national press that are relevant in advance

- If you can, try to swing one of the other two styles into this one – choosing a topic you are totally confident with

Aggressive/closed questions

17

In this chapter

- How do you prepare for hostile questioning?
- What is the interviewer trying to achieve by this method?
- How can you turn a very negative situation into a strong selling position?

This is the most feared type of interview: where your decisions and motivations are picked apart and criticised. Often, the way you handle a hypothetical situation that hasn't even yet arisen is the source of the aggressive question.

As with open/retrospective questioning, you will be warned that this style is being used by the candidates ahead of you. Here they tend to come out looking more stressed than when they went in and say 'they were really nasty' or 'I didn't have a chance to say anything to them, they just seemed to want to attack me'. Usually, the interpretation they put on this is that they have not been successful.

This style is not the most difficult type of interview. Certainly the interviewers might be nasty to you or seem not to be listening. But you are practically given the opportunity to sell yourself on a plate. And there is no chance whatsoever of seeming arrogant.

The aim of polishing technique with this style is to get beyond the affect used by the interviewer. Because it is a reasonable bet that everyone else is being given the same treatment you have a huge advantage if you understand how to deal with it.

BASIC PRINCIPLES

Under pressure

This is a style that is really only testing one aspect of your readiness for the job: your ability to cope under pressure. The questions openly and unremittingly put you under increasing pressure. The assumption is that the best candidate will be able to cope with the pressure of the interview. And that is – probably erroneously – linked in the interviewer's mind with an ability to do the job that is on offer.

Feels like a television interview

It is exactly the same style as used by combative journalists, particularly when interviewing politicians. Often confusing the sheer unremitting nature of their questions with an effective interview, these interviewers aim to extract 'confessions' from their guests – confessions, perhaps of a policy or personal failure, that would not be made without unrelenting pressure of this kind.

Always focused on the failures

So the style is all about failure. It is negative, critical and devastatingly effective in destroying a candidate's morale, by cruelly exposing all your failures and missed opportunities, and situations where you simply didn't do well enough.

Seeks broad examples

Often, the questions will relate to unconnected incidents or events in the past, seeking to demonstrate a track-record of disasters, and crystal-ball-gazing as to how you would perform in some hypothetical situation in your future life. And your non-medical

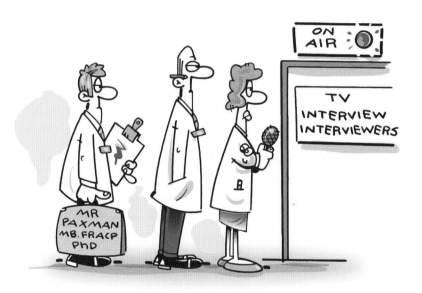

An aggressive interviewing style

life might also be drawn into the interview (most commonly by you).

RECOGNISING THE STYLE

This is the easiest style to recognise because it is always launched into. You can almost imagine the interviewer psyching up beforehand, practising the delivery of the first knock-out blow to perfection.

Questions are delivered quickly and forcefully, and you are often interrupted halfway through, implying a lack of interest in the answer. The topic might be changed abruptly. The situations that are used in this style hover between the past, present and future.

Top Tip
Questions are often not specifically phrased to ask about work situations and you can often use non-work examples, such as from extra-curricular or your home life to answer. This has the advantage of being much less easy for the interviewer to criticise because it is more personal.

Comparison between questions in open/retrospective and aggressive/closed styles:

	Open/retrospective	Aggressive/closed
Length	Longer	Shorter
Balance of talking	With interviewee	With interviewer
Temporal relationship of questions	Always in the past	Mixture of past and future
Question stem	Vague, broad	Precise, narrow
Person discussed in interview topic	Always you	May be others, or a mixture

COMMON PITFALLS

Too rehearsed

Many interview candidates prepare and rehearse the answers to these questions, and many more hypothetical ones, by rote. It is easy for experienced interviewers to tell when answers have been practised and it tends to lead to more difficult and more aggressive supplementals.

Matching the anger

When someone is aggressive towards you, you get stressed and your chest tightens with frustration. There is no doubt this style of questioning *is* frustrating. But you have to accept – as in all interviews – that the panel is in charge. If the panel members want to ask aggressive question after aggressive question, that is up to them. You might find yourself resenting it and getting angry but matching the interviewer's anger is the wrong thing to do. You are being tested on your ability to cope with pressure and if the panel members see you cracking up they might assume that is the way you always behave when you are up against it. You are rejected for this reason alone. Whatever happens, and however frustrated you feel, do not get angry.

Too confident

Candidates who are experienced interviewees may have been presented with similar lists of questions many times. SHOs who interview for 10 different rotations might get broadly similar aggressive/closed questions on each occasion.

By the time you have been asked the same questions so many times it is very easy to start to anticipate the questions. In other words, you know that a certain question is coming up and you jump into the answer without thinking about it. But, psychologically, when the questioner is anticipating that the question stem is a difficult one (i.e. aggressive/closed), this reaction makes you seem overconfident. This can also prevent you from getting the job.

Repeating yourself

In this respect, this style is the same as the open/retrospective style.

It is easy to have thought of only one or two examples to illustrate weaknesses or failings. And if the questions go on and on in the same vein it can be a real challenge to come up with more examples that you can use. Candidates frequently repeat examples ('As I said previously...'), which is poor technique because it implies that you think you have only one weakness or failing in your life.

Top Tip
Again, don't forget you can always bring in non-work examples with this style.

COMMON QUESTIONS

'What is your greatest weakness?'

This is the most common question asked in medical interviews: it is even more common than the open/retrospective question 'Why do you want the job?' It is the most popular, most predictable, and most trite question asked.

In one sense, the question is reasonable. Recognising weaknesses is an important part of career development. Openness about areas that need developing is vital to organisational success and motivating teams. Weaknesses require work, or expose a flank that might need to be covered by a colleague or another member of the team.

The problem with the question is that is has become self-perpetuating. Because everyone knows it is coming, it is the most prepared question before the interview and therefore the answer sounds like it is being read off a teleprompter. It therefore has no discriminatory value. Better interviewers avoid the question for this reason.

 Don't be too rehearsed with this question. Everybody gives the answer about being too diligent or 'a perfectionist' because they think it implies that they are a caring doctor. Some panels have told me that every single candidate gave the same reply. Be original with your answer and not a perfectionist!

Other common questions

- The other candidates outside are better than you. What should we say to them if we gave the post to you?
- How do you handle rejection?
- Your consultant is making lots of bizarre decisions that don't seem to conform with good medical practice. What do you do about it?
- Have you always followed evidence-based medicine?
- How do we know you would be a good member of the team?
- How do you demonstrate leadership?
- When was the last time you didn't get on with one of your colleagues and how did you deal with that?
- We don't think you are qualified enough for the job so why should we give it to you?
- When have you failed in your career?
- What are the most disappointing points of your career so far?
- If you retired at 65, under what situation would you feel you had failed your career ambitions?
- Does anyone think you are going to get this job?

- When was the last time your work was criticised and how do you deal with that?
- If a colleague on the rotation began to take drugs what would you do about it?
- If one of your co-SHOs was not performing adequately what would you say to them?

POLISHING TECHNIQUE

Learning from the past

Past failings and weaknesses are something that we all have, and being able to discuss these is an important part of developing both individually and professionally. But the key is that we learnt from the mistakes of the past and that they won't be repeated.

Finding the positives

It is widely known that the trick to these questions is to be able to turn the weakness, or the negative situation, to your advantage. You are suggesting you are a better person because of the insight you have into the previous situation. Although this is part of the technique, you have to make sure to include enough of the learning element as well. In effect, good technique is summarised as:

- What did you learn from in the past?
- How have you behaved differently since?

The best answers reflect both of these two stages.

Practise being challenged

Get someone to throw a series of aggressive questions at you and practise the feeling of being put on the spot. Watch one of the more aggressive television interviewers and see how they do it.

Make sure that you sell yourself through the answer, without being too defensive, and:

- don't match the aggression
- don't let the interviewer destroy your confidence.

Don't repeat examples

Poor interviewees constantly repeat the same example in answer to all sorts of different, aggressive question stems. The panel will assume you have insight into only one of your failings, and therefore aren't aware of all the others. When preparing, think of lots of different illustrations and introduce them sequentially as needed.

Non-medical examples

This is the best style of interview into which to introduce examples of when you learnt from your past in a non-medical sphere of life. Whether from medical school, extra-curricular life, committee or community work, family life or anything else. This is great technique for two reasons:

- It is much harder for the panel members to be critical of your non-medical 'errors' because they might come across as being biased.
- They know nothing about the situation and so cannot be too challenging.

Don't rehearse answers by rote

As mentioned before, this is the style where a well-prepared candidate with poor technique sticks out like a sore thumb. It is really tempting to learn answers to the most common of these questions by heart. But the panel can easily tell. Instead, think about the general topics you want to bring up, and the way in which you are going to come across. Be reflective and thoughtful about your past.

Summary

- This style is also known as the 'they were so horrible' style

- Despite the open aggression, it is easy to sell yourself

- When answering, try to come across as being open and reflective, and pepper the interview with as many non-medical situations as you can think of

18

Specific types of medical job application

In this chapter

- How do you prepare for academic job interviews?
- New styles of selection – how do you prepare for:
  - presentations?
  - OSCE-style interviews?
  - written answer assessments?

ACADEMIC JOBS

All jobs in clinical medicine are assessed in part from an academic perspective. Academic qualifications, expertise and authority are not bad things. They indicate curiousness and an ability to follow well-established scientific methodology to achieve greater knowledge. And ultimately it is the best of the academic physicians who contribute most to medical breakthroughs.

But most clinicians don't want to be academics. My work with consultants has allowed me to formulate a clear distinction between the two types. First, those who want senior lectureships with an honourary consultant contract (i.e. academic physicians) and second, those who want substantive consultant positions, with a varying element of teaching and research.

The majority are in the second group – including almost all in district general hospitals and more than half in teaching hospitals.

The problem is that doctors in training feel obliged to develop academic credentials even if they have no interest in pursuing academic careers; GPs don't have any such requirements. Our analysis indicated a fascination, bordering on the obsessive, with academic track record. And interview questions tend to follow suit in including heavy bias towards academic success.

This section is specifically tailored to those positions that are academic:

- research posts
- fellowships linked to research
- attachments to research and academic units where part of the role involves research
- university appointments for clinicians.

THE CV AND APPLICATION FORM

In the written parts of the application the need to sell an academic track record is absolutely paramount. In this situation, the needs of the buyers are absolutely specific. They are buying a past performer in academia who will perform for them. I live in a family of academics and the requirements for academic success were the staple diet of the dinner table.

PAPER QUALIFICATIONS

Make the academic qualifications central: they are your big hitters and must be placed high up the CV, and to the left of the page. And as always, it is *what* followed by *where* followed by *when*, so:

First class honours BSc → University of London → 1996

Ask the expert

Can I apply for an academic post without any academic credentials?

You would be starting from a low point but you do have two options. First, you have to be able to sell complementary skills and accomplishments. Have you shown an interest in publications, presentations, etc.? Second, you should ask a buyer whether they would consider an application.

Academic prizes are also big hitters in academic CVs and should be treated as such.

PUBLICATIONS

The way to set out publications was discussed in Chapter 5. If you have a great number, append them to the CV as a bibliography.

It is important that the outcome of research – if not apparent from the title of the paper – is made clear. Later on, the ability to get articles accepted by major peer-reviewed journals is important because it forms part of the university Research Assessment Exercise (RAE).

PRESENTATIONS

These tend to be useful earlier on in academic careers and less so later on. For medical students, PRHOs and early-stage SHOs, the opportunity for papers and certainly higher degrees might not exist. But you still have to demonstrate some commitment to academia and useful presentations might be the answer.

Don't belittle the academically focused presentations by also including presentations to the rugby club on funding issues. Remember the needs of the buyer: it isn't that the latter presentation wasn't a success, it is that these buyers are interested in academic presentations, and not the others.

THE INTERVIEW

An understanding of scientific methodology will be expected. Statistical analysis forms part of this and is often something that candidates don't prepare for. When revising your big hitters for the open/retrospective questions, demonstrate the outcomes of your research. In particular, what happened after you finished a specific project: did the research continue and in what way were your conclusions built upon?

Occasionally, you might be asked to bring your papers to interview: check if this is the case and get them ready in good time. Well-presented, original off-prints are much better than photocopies but need some planning to collect for interviews.

INTERVIEWS WITH 'BOLT-ONS'

Three trends have emerged in recent years in the development of the medical selection process:

- a presentation component to the interview
- OSCE-style interviews
- a written component.

Presentations

It is beyond the scope of this book to cover presentation skills in detail. When required as part of the interview stage of medical job applications, there are a number of basic principles:

- The presentation is always short.
- It tends to be on a management issue, such as planning services, or of problem-solving nature, rather than a straight clinical scenario.
- It is usually required at the same time as the interview: so you need to be able to switch from the presentation to the interview quickly.

 Remember that the panel will have asked for the same presentation from every candidate who has been shortlisted. Particularly if the topic is an obvious one, try to think of ways of livening up your presentation. Otherwise there is a risk of the panel being bored to death. In this case your interview might start on a bad footing and rapidly deteriorate.

General considerations
Timing:

- Hopefully, the overall timings of the presentation will be given to you.
- If it is not, assume a presentation of no more than 5 minutes.
- Emerging questions are a likely kick-start for the rest of the interview.
- Under no circumstances exceed the time allotted.

Visual aids:

- PowerPoint might not be available: check before preparing slides.
- Remember that good visual aids are not the same as a good presentation.
- Consider producing a 1-page handout summarising the main points, which can be given to the panel before you start speaking.

OSCE-style interviews

Objective structured clinical examinations (OSCEs) have been proven repeatedly to be more sensitive and specific in testing clinical skills than long and short cases. As a result, they are the norm now in clinical examinations at every stage of medical training. Every medical school and postgraduate college examination uses the OSCE format.

OSCE-style interviews have been introduced at pilot stage in many Trusts and form the major form of selection in many more. There are several advantages and disadvantages of this format:

Advantages of OSCE format	Disadvantages of OSCE format
More objective	Much more time consuming
Allows candidates to perform badly in one or more stations but still be more successful	Tends to be a disadvantage for candidates good at formal interviews as other styles are tested
Greater range of interview styles tested	Organisationally complex and requires many more 'interviewers'
Transparency of process reassuring to both candidates and interviewers	More expensive
Reproducible every time the job is readvertised with few changes	Interviewers cannot explore issues in as much depth as required: tends to lead to a more superficial interview

The interviewee proceeds around a time-limited series of stations where a pair of interviewers alternatively ask questions and mark answers. At the end, the marks are totalled and the candidates with the best scores are offered the jobs.

Because of the complexity of organising OSCE interviews they are much more commonly used for rotations where several appointments begin concurrently. It is beyond the needs of stand-alone jobs to organise an OSCE.

Top Tip
Normally in interviews clinical acumen is not part of the assessment. But here expect one or more clinical stations. Examples in OSCEs I have been involved with include communication skills, resuscitation and clinical problem solving.

Most of the OSCE stations will include one or two of the questions divided up between the information in Chapters 15, 16 and 17. Your answers might be written down formally. One station will be based around your answer to just one question. There is little chance for you, the interviewee, to influence the direction of the interview.

Ask the expert
Should I prepare differently if I find out the interview is OSCE based?
No, but do remember that clinical scenarios might be introduced. Think about relevant scenarios and add these into the preparation. All the interview questions are identical to those covered earlier and should be prepared for in the same way.

Written answers

This is not the same as the 'personal statement', which might be included on an application form and is part of shortlisting. This written answer stage is post-shortlisting.

The written answer has also been introduced for pre-medical school application. It forms part of the Graduate Australian Medical School Admission Test (GAMSAT) examination that is widely used to select postgraduate medical students. And as entry for undergraduate students becomes more competitive, and more candidates obtain the highest possible A-level grades, other selection tools have been brought in. As well as psychometrics, the written answer is becoming common.

The main difference is that at the medical school admission level the subject matter is normally logic and argument. For instance:

'Medicine is more an art than a science.' Do you agree?

Written answers at job selection are similar to the subjects chosen for the formal presentation. Management, service provision and problem solving are more common than clinical scenarios. I haven't heard of an example of the GAMSAT-style of question being used.

General principles

- If it is a typed answer, sign it at the bottom to make it clear it is your work.
- Observe the set word limit. Preferably stick to one side of A4.
- If you give opinions, make sure you acknowledge the other side of the argument (see Chapter 17).
- Use short, succinct sentences and bullets where possible, remembering you are going for easy readability because the assessor might spend very little time on your reply.

Finally, bear in mind that the written answer is only part of the assessment and do not neglect the other components of your preparation.

19

Closing the interview and following up

- How to conclude the interview on a positive note?
- What should you expect next?
- What can you do if you aren't successful?

ANYTHING TO ASK US?

This is usually the last question posed and it is another trick question. I'll explain why. There is almost no question you can ask that will improve your chances of getting the job.

If you think about it, they are asking this last question of you because they have completed the interview. The decision has already been made whether you have been successful or not. Either you've got the job or you haven't.

If you have been successful at this stage there is no point in asking any questions. The only possible outcome is that they change their minds because you ask a stupid question.

If you have not got the job, theoretically you could get them to change their minds in your favour by asking a brilliant question. But I have never heard a brilliant question asked.

There are lots of bad questions to ask, which may be summarised.

- Relating information you should already have got:

'What are my responsibilities when on call?'
'Do I work for Dr Smith on a Monday'
'Do I have the opportunity for a colorectal clinic?'

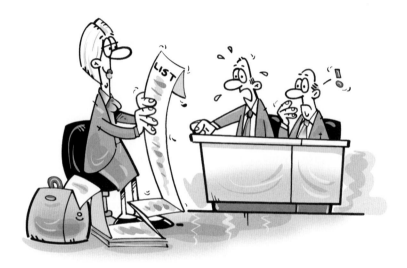

'Have you anything to ask us?

Asking any of these questions implies you have not researched the job terribly well – if you've got the job they might change their minds.

● Facile questions to which the answer is always 'yes':

'Are there opportunities for research/teaching/audit work/presentations?'
'Do you encourage your SHO to . . .?'
'Would you support me in sitting the MRCS/applying for SpR posts?'

Asking these questions implies you are crawling: not necessary if you have got the job and pointless if you haven't.

Top Tip
Don't ask a question at the end. Politely say you have nothing to ask and get out of there as quickly as possible.

FINISHING THE INTERVIEW

The process of leaving the interview panel is described in Chapter 14. Shake hands only if offered but smile at the panel, thank them for their time and leave confidently – even if you are absolutely sure you haven't been successful. Don't forget that the aggressive/closed interview style can come across as having gone very badly when in fact it hasn't.

Don't be tempted to give other candidates a run-down of the questions. You only help them as they then have time to prepare when you did not. Don't help them. Remember they will most likely be given the same questions as you did. Leave the waiting room immediately and go for a walk and get a coffee instead.

GOOD NEWS: YOU'VE BEEN SUCCESSFUL

Accepting the job

The chair of the panel will tell you when the decision will be made and if you are likely to have to commit yourself to accepting it straight away. There are three possibilities:

1. You will be informed as soon as all the interviews are over and the panel has had a final discussion (often at 7 or 8 in the evening).
2. You will be informed by telephone, or can phone the HR department on a certain day to get the result.
3. You will be informed by letter of the decision.

In the first instance you might have to accept straight away. Often, the successful interviewees are called first and offered the jobs. If any turn the job down then further interviewees might be asked if they will take the job, until all the posts are filled.

Ask the expert

Can I ask for a delay in giving an answer to the panel in the event of being expected to accept the job immediately? Many people would give an emphatic negative answer to this. But consultants sometimes try to bully people into accepting a job straight away. You could try to ask for a compromise any reasonable individual would accept: such as a 24-hour delay. And give a good reason: you need to relocate your family and must discuss it with them. The panel is trying to avoid being messed about by individual doctors who are juggling lots of jobs and, to be fair to the recruiters, they do have to ensure jobs are filled and need a commitment from you at some time. But don't be afraid to ask for a reasonable delay.

The latter two situations require you to accept the job formally in writing, or to telephone. You always have a delay and can therefore make the decision whether to take the job.

 Top Tip
If you can, decide whether you would accept the job if offered on the day of the interview. This saves any embarrassment on either side.

Other issues to consider before beginning the job

You might need to clarify:

- Whether any paperwork is needed from you by the Trust before you start work.
- If your salary needs clarifying before signing a contract.
- How long the job is for.

BAD NEWS: YOU HAVE NOT BEEN SUCCESSFUL

Failing to get a job is always deflating. It's worse at this stage than failing to be shortlisted because so much more work has gone into the process. And you have expended a huge amount of emotional energy on the day itself.

The premise of the whole of this book is to make you feel positive, to allow for honing of technique and to try to get you to believe you can be successful. But it might not happen. I haven't ever met a consultant who succeeded at each interview attempt. Failing to get a job isn't a prerequisite for a career not going well: quite the opposite. And there are lots and lots of jobs. So what should you do if you aren't successful?

Write down the questions

On the train home, list all the questions you were asked and what your answers (in outline) were. You won't remember the following day. It is important to be able to review your answers critically before the next interview. But don't assume you answered anything wrongly. It could have been that your confidence or technique was poor, rather than your answers. And there could have been a superb candidate who blew everyone else away.

Take the night off

It's easy to mope on a bad day and I do it as much as anyone else. But take the night off: don't agree to cover someone else's night shift. Have a meal out and watch a movie, try to relax. It's sometimes difficult to remember that tomorrow is another day.

Get feedback

This is great in principle but rarely helpful in practice. Corporate recruiters are excellent at providing structured, useful feedback to unsuccessful candidates. Headhunters are even better. But consultants and other medical recruiters are dreadful at it. The most common feedback people report to me is 'You were good but we had a slightly better candidate'. That's English for crawling off the hook. It is hopeless for the candidate and it gives no chance to learn from the experience.

You need to avoid a totally open question like 'Please can I have some feedback?' because you might end up with the answer above.

 Top Tip
Prepare a set of questions before asking for feedback. Consider asking for clarification of answers you didn't know during the interview. Or for their reaction to answers you gave. The more closed your questions, the easier for the interviewer to help you. At all costs avoid 'Please can I have some feedback?'

Stay positive

Easier said than done. But you have got to get a job and getting deflated won't improve your performance. Write a list of the things to improve on for next time, and of the topics you were asked that you didn't know or didn't perform well on. And concentrate on getting these answers sorted before the next interview. Try not to ruminate on what happened too much, it might be you never work out why you weren't successful.

Interview practice

It is possible to organise practice, and often people come to me saying they have been recommended by an interview panel to get some practice. It is important to try to follow the suggestion with a more closed question such as:

> 'What aspects of my performance do I specifically need to get interview practice on?'

Not only does this focus your preparation for the next interview but helps anyone who is going to coach you.

Summary

- Don't ask questions at the end of the interview: just thank the panel and leave

- If successful, make sure you decide whether to accept the job in advance

- If unsuccessful, remember that tomorrow is another day and, when getting feedback, make it specific by asking closed questions of the panel

Summary of interviews

20

In this chapter

- How do typical medical interviews proceed?

- What are the most common pitfalls to be aware of?

- How do you work out how to hone your personal technique using the hints in the previous chapters?

COMBINATION INTERVIEWS

Interview questions are split into three styles:

1. open/retrospective
2. topical
3. aggressive/closed.

All interview questions can be fitted into one of these categories. But it is not true that the whole interview is just of one of these styles. Most commonly the questions switch from one style to another, quite randomly, and then back again.

Let's say that one of the consultants has been asked to concentrate on clinical governance and audit, one of the most common topics. This person could actually use any of the styles to question the candidates, or a mixture of all of them, so:

- 'Tell me about your experiences of clinical audit' (open/retrospective)
- 'You don't seem to have much experience of audit work' (aggressive/closed)
- 'What do you understand about the principles of audit' (topical).

Every potential interview topic can be thought of in the same way.

Top Tip
When preparing for your interview, try to think of ways in which the same topic could be questioned in each of the three styles. That way you will prepare you answers accordingly.

When you think of the interview in this way, the difference between the open/retrospective and aggressive/closed styles could not be clearer:

'Tell me about your experiences of clinical audit.'

- Sounds friendly and relaxing, a 'they were so nice' kind of question.
- You could waffle on for hours.
- You might end up selling someone else's audit ability (like the professor, who is quite capable of selling himself).

'You don't seem to have much experience of audit work.'

- Puts you on the defensive, 'they were so horrible'.
- Tends to make you fight your corner: in other words to sell yourself.
- Will probably be interrupted with another question before you have gone on for too long.

MOVING FROM STYLE TO STYLE

If the panel is switching rapidly between styles, you might end up feeling as if you can't follow the direction the interview is going.

In these circumstances it is vital to pause and think before you start the answer.

Don't think you have understood the question? Make sure you have understood it before attempting an answer. You can't ask for a clarification once you have started replying.

Before answering a question, work out which of the three styles it is. Then remember the key points of selling yourself from each style (see Chapters 15, 16 and 17). Don't attempt to rush into an answer. Make sure you have thought through the reason for asking the question first.

Top Tip
Behind every question is a point; questions are not asked for no reason. As the salesman sitting in front of the buyers, it is essential to work out what they are looking to purchase in giving your answer.

MOST COMMON PITFALLS TO AVOID IN ALL STYLES OF INTERVIEW

What should I do if there are long pauses in the interview?

Nothing. Don't try to fill the silences because you will waffle on. You can only sell yourself effectively if you know what the buyers want to buy. You can only find this out by dissecting and analysing their questions. A monologue won't help you at all. Wait for them to ask the next question.

What if one of the panel leaves during the interview or someone arrives?

Don't forget this is their interview and they control the rules. You might think them rude but just carry on and don't get too flustered. Do not attempt to talk to the newcomer: if the chair wants your points to be summarised you will be asked to do so. If someone has left, it is a safe bet that person will not be responsible for the decision at the end of the session.

What should I do if offered a cup of tea?

Never forget that your nerves can be controlled but your hands give them away. It isn't possible to drink from a glass or cup without the cup shaking if you are nervous. No beverages.

What if I don't have an answer to a question?

In topical questions this might not be a problem, and you should never say you know about something if you don't. The panel ought to move on. But repeated 'I don't knows' are likely to leave them cold. In open/retrospective and aggressive/closed styles you should probably have an answer to all the questions. Ask for a moment to think and gather your thoughts if you need to.

What if I am constantly interrupted?

Most likely you are in an aggressive/closed interview and this is part of the style. Everyone is getting the same treatment. Remember to sell your successes and always try to turn the negatives into positives, demonstrating what you have learnt over your career.

What if I can tell they aren't going to give me the job?

You might be right. Rudeness on the part of the panel, as distinct from an aggressive question, might be the clue. Don't get angry, after all there is nothing you can do about it.

HONING YOUR PERSONAL TECHNIQUE: TEN LAST TIPS

Really good interview technique is built by remembering:

1. There is no such thing as a perfect interview answer and under no circumstances should you rote-learn answers as a way of getting through the interview: you will be spotted instantly.

2. You can always improve answers. Practising different stems, such as to the audit question above, is helpful in predicting the types of question that will arise.

3. Whenever a story about the medical world, or the NHS, appears in the media stop and think what the two sides of the argument are: this will prepare you for the topical questions.

4. The interview is all about sales and you should consider your preparation in terms of identifying what the buyers are in the market to buy.

5. It is just as important to be able to get on with the panel members as to be the best candidate available: they have to work with you when they have given you the job.

6. Try to work out what doubts the interviewer will have about you and slay them before a question is asked about these doubts, if possible.

7. Moving the interviewer onto a 'good' topic for you is always great technique.

8. In general, if you are well prepared the topical style will score you most points.

9. It is always a competitive process: don't give your competitors any information that might help them. Don't give them any at all; keep them guessing.

10. If you try to enjoy yourself you will appear relaxed and confident.

Top Tip
Never stop selling your achievements. Read and reread your big hitters and make sure you sell them effectively. Hone your sales into what the specific buyers on the other side of the table seem to want and do your homework to try to predict this.

Summary

- Remember that all potential subjects can be introduced in each of the three styles of interview question: think of ways of rephrasing questions to fit each type

- Beware of irritating problems that occur, and don't forget – no beverages!

- As the last thought, never forget that it's all about selling yourself – again and again – if you want the job

General practice

There is no fundamental difference between applying for hospital jobs and GP jobs. All GP careers begin in hospital medicine and at these stages the application and interview process is identical. But there are some differences in approach and, when applying for a substantive partnership or salaried post, the process is different.

WHAT'S DIFFERENT?

Currently, there are two ways of gaining training towards accreditation for general practice. This accreditation is called a vocational training number (VTN), and is required for substantive GP posts. The main feature is that training to become a GP is many years shorter because the registrar stage is one year, compared with five years for hospital posts. There is also much less need to take time out of the training years for research.

1. Vocational training schemes (VTS)

These are geared specifically towards the requirements of the VTN award. As with hospital training posts, the regionally based Deaneries control access to these jobs, and they oversee the suitability of individual jobs to be 'counted' towards the VTN award.

Various hospital specialties are linked to form a bedrock of suitable experience. Medicine, paediatrics, obstetrics and gynaecology and psychiatry might be linked together for instance. Applicants for VTS schemes will typically expect to work in four different hospital subspecialties over two years.

At the end of the initial two-year period a further 'GP Registrar' year is linked to the VTS, normally without further application. So, unlike hospital-based specialist registrars, there is no need for further interview at this stage.

2. Stand-alone schemes

As with hospital jobs, an alternative is to create an individually tailored GP training programme, remembering that this must be agreed by the local Deanery to be considered appropriate. Reasons for this approach might be:

- The local VTS doesn't include the range of specialties you wish to cover.
- You want to spend more than six months in one specialty, for instance, if you have a particular interest in paediatrics you might wish to spend a year on it.
- You initially began training in hospital medicine (for instance in paediatrics or general medicine) and decide to switch.

SWITCHING INTO GENERAL PRACTICE TRAINING

This is not normally difficult. Many SHOs decide after a year or more of their hospital training that a career in general practice would be more suitable. It would be incredibly unlucky if at least some of your jobs are not counted for the VTN. The Royal College of General Practitioners website provides information on the principles of conversion, and the local Deanery would need to be contacted on your specific situation (see Appendix 2).

At the stage of deciding to convert into general practice you have two options:

- Apply for a VTS.
- Continue to 'add on' further stand-alone six month jobs to complete the hospital stage of the VTN requirements.

In the case of stand-alone rotations it is possible to qualify for a VTN by completing just three jobs over two years. One job can last one year and then continue with two different six-month jobs. So if you have completed one year of general medicine it would be normal just to have to choose two different specialties to complete the requirements.

GP REGISTRAR YEAR

What is different, however, with the stand-alone approach is that you have to apply for GP registrar posts in isolation. Remember that in the VTS this year is included. Deaneries provide lists of training practices that offer GP registrar posts on a stand-alone basis. The jobs are advertised in *BMJ Careers* in the normal way.

SUBSTANTIVE GP POSTS

Currently, GP posts are available on a salaried or partnered basis. The interview process is different from most hospital positions in that it is much more unpredictable because it is carried out by the current GPs at the practice to which you are applying. Only GPs, and sometimes the practice manager, are involved with the process. The wide-ranging panels, including hospital management and lay representatives, that are typical in hospital appointments, do not happen here. Some practices like to conduct part of the selection process informally, over lunch or dinner, and 'trial by sherry' is therefore more commonly part of the decision.

Any occasion where you meet the prospective colleagues at a new GP practice is part of the selection process. Don't drop your guard just because the interview is at someone's house or at a restaurant.

This more uncertain approach doesn't change the principles of interviewing. But without HR departments watching the procedure it is more difficult to predict the outcome. And GPs who are less experienced at interviewing have a tendency to want to employ someone like them, rather than someone who complements the team and adds to it.

TOPICAL INTERVIEW QUESTIONS

Expect questions relating to current affairs and trends in GP management, training and continual professional development. Current hot topics include:

- Employment arrangements for GPs relating to contracts.
- Partnerships versus salaried GPs.
- Employment of non-traditional therapists in GP surgeries.
- Training format, including input into medical student teaching.
- Guidelines and targets.
- Computerisation of records and practice information.
- Continuous professional development, including quality and practice audit.
- Primary care trusts and their relationship with the practices.
- Subspecialisation of GPs.
- Local clinics where consultants are contracted to work in the PCT for a set period per week.

Doctor magazine, published weekly by Reed Business Press and available free of charge, is the best place to find out which issues are in current debate.

Summary

- The basic principles of completing a CV and interviewing are the same for all jobs in medicine

- The major difference is at the final stage, when interviews are more unpredictable because they are organised by individual GP practices

- Topical questions are best prepared with review of the GP-specific press but would also include wider NHS and political issues

Assessment tools

22

- What other methods of selection are available apart from the CV and interview?
- What is psychometric testing and what is its objective?
- If a selection tool is being applied to an application, how do you prepare for it?

Twenty-five years ago, selection for jobs across the workforce in the UK was by CV, shortlist to interview and job offer. In the medical profession this is still by far the most common pattern. But the wider recruitment world has realised that, because the job market has changed fundamentally, there is a need to alter the way in which selection for roles is undertaken.

Selection tools have already been introduced at medical school admission stage and psychometric testing has been used extensively in career-choice planning, most specifically at SHO level. So it seems fairly sure that part of the recruitment process will include assessment tools in the future. And all readers who are considering applying for non-NHS jobs using their medical degree can expect these tests as a matter of routine.

WHY ARE ASSESSMENT TOOLS USED?

To assess fit

It is really important for organisations to ensure that new hires will fit in with the culture and 'feel' it has created. No company with an open, non-hierarchical culture would want to employ Captain Mainwaring from *Dad's Army*, for instance.

To help choose the best candidate

Many interview panels conclude with a dead heat between suitable candidates. This is unsatisfying for both the unsuccessful candidates and the panel – who wonder for the rest of the rotation if they have chosen the right person. So an assessment tool might be used to help make the decision.

To be objective

As discussed repeatedly through the book, interviews are an incredibly subjective process. Many interviewers are still guilty of choosing the candidate most like them rather than the best candidate.

WHAT KINDS OF ASSESSMENT TOOLS ARE THERE?

A number of different tools are available; some have more relevance than others. But for completeness they are all described. Numerical reasoning:

- basic arithmetic to ensure numeracy
- data interpretation
- problem solving, such as straightforward algebra.

Verbal reasoning:

- spelling: frequently the identification of misspelled words in a list
- word meaning: synonyms and antonyms
- verbal comprehension: how words are being used.

Abstract reasoning:

- looking at series of symbols and analysing patterns.

Perceptual reasoning:

- information is presented in diagrammatic form
- popular because doesn't require good working knowledge of English

- examples include clock faces and arrows that present information.

Spatial reasoning:

- interpretation and manipulation of two-dimensional figures.

PERSONALITY TESTING (PSYCHOMETRICS)

Principles of psychometric testing

Psychometrics is a huge topic and the subject of much research and even more controversy. Detailed information is available from many good sources (see Appendix 3).

Individuals answer questions on their preferences, feelings, behaviours and motivations. This information is then analysed, in part by electronic means and in part by specialist interpreters, to try to tease out patterns. The results should then always be followed by an in-depth interview to check the patterns are correct and to challenge the results as needed. Psychometric testing as a 'cold', computerised exercise can be more harmful than helpful because the results need careful and specialised interpretation.

The most well-known psychometric testing is the Myers–Briggs indicator, which profiles individuals on four scales:

E/I   extroverted/introverted
S/I   sensing/intuitive
T/F   thinking/feeling
J/P   judging/perceiving.

These scales try to place individuals somewhere on a line between two opposites, and this position is then used to predict likely responses to situations. There isn't a right or wrong profile and it is very dangerous to read too much into the answers without being put into context.

Don't try to prepare set answers thinking that an employer is looking for a specific personality type. The test asks repeated questions in slightly different ways and mixes up answers and the interpreter will be able to detect your attempt to produce a different personality than the true one.

There is a big difference between psychometrics and 360-degree evaluation testing (see below). Psychometrics is always based on your own interpretation of your behaviour. Although your friends think you are extroverted, you might perceive yourself as introverted and the results of the test will reflect this. Psychometrics is, by definition, not done on your behalf by your friends.

360-DEGREE EVALUATION

This is a complementary form of assessment. You have no input into it at all. Your colleagues, friends, manager, trainer, trainees, and even patients, assess your personality. They are asked detailed questions about your effectiveness and behaviour and these are then interpreted to give an overall picture. This is especially effective in leadership development, where it is widely and successfully used.

The '360' bit implies that it isn't an appraisal, where one person gives an opinion on you, but involves people from all over your spectrum of work. Importantly, it isn't just your boss but also colleagues who report into you in some way who are asked.

So a typical 360-degree evaluation for a medical SHO might involve:

- their consultant
- their PRHO
- their medical student
- a nurse in outpatients

- a nurse or doctor in A&E
- someone in a completely different department (such as radiology) with which they work
- one or more patients who have been treated by the individual.

The big disadvantage of 360-degree assessment is that it is time consuming and therefore managerially expensive to carry out. Psychometrics is relatively quick and cheap.

IN-TRAY EXERCISES

These are tests of managing time and prioritisation. Essentially, a theoretical in-tray is created and you are tested on your ability to manage the information provided.

Assume, for instance, you have just got out of clinic and you have seven bleeps to answer, a note to contact the departmental secretary urgently, a patient has complained about something, and your PRHO has decided to quit the job. You only have an hour before you have to be in theatre. The idea is to test how you manage this information, analyse it and prioritise your responses.

Practical, realistic and objective, in-tray exercises are good assessments and will become much more a part of selection and development within the medical profession.

PREPARING FOR ASSESSMENT EXERCISES

You will be informed of the type of exercise that is going to be employed but you might not be clear as to exactly which types of reasoning tests are included. There are many books available with practice tests to give you some idea – kept in the management sections of the bookshop. I know people who have prepared for the verbal reasoning testing by learning 20 new words from the dictionary every day, which is one way of building vocabulary. Mental arithmetic is something that is probably more innate than taught. And certainly you shouldn't try to prepare too hard for psychometric testing.

The only really good advice is to be alert and ready for the test and, as with all examinations, watch the time carefully. Don't agree to attend an assessment exercise the morning after a night shift. And don't overanalyse what you are being asked to do.

Sometimes the tests can actually be quite fun.

Summary

- If an assessment tool is introduced it can be thought of as either some sort of reasoning, or a psychometric assessment

- Reasoning tests can be prepared for but psychometrics is an assessment of insight into personality and therefore cannot

- Don't be afraid of these assessments, which are only part of any application process: good interview technique is still vital

23

The future of medical selection

In this chapter

- What are the trends within medical selection currently?
- What is driving these trends?
- How is the selection process likely to change in the next few years?

The major criticism of the current selection process is that it is biased and unfair. Bias is introduced at almost every stage, and is very difficult to eliminate. The readers of a CV can, as we have shown, be influenced by a well-presented document that adequately sells the candidate. The interview is not normally recorded and so queries and discrepancies and complaints cannot be checked. And ultimately the panel can ask absolutely anything it wants.

As one small example, Professor Ian McManus proved, in seminal work from the 1980s, that medical school selection panels were racially biased. The effect of his work was to remove personal identifying details from applications to medical schools in an attempt to eliminate this. Currently this isn't done at post-qualification level.

Delegates from outside the UK are disadvantaged in a number of ways:

- The process takes place in English, which might not be the first language.
- Written English – such as on an application form – is very different from the spoken format of an interview.

- Overseas qualifications, awards and other achievements might not be recognised by selectors and therefore the candidate does not get shortlisted.

But it isn't just non-UK candidates that might not be treated equally. Conclusions are drawn from all sorts of information on applications that is not relevant to the candidate's ability to do the job. I am horrified by the number of women, and increasingly men, who are knocked back because they took career breaks.

A number of trends have emerged over the past couple of years:

- increased use of non-medical, and particularly non-consultant, interviewers
- far more training of interviewers in good technique
- introduction of more than one interview (such as an OSCE)
- presentations and written answers
- psychometric assessments as part of the process.

DRIVERS FOR CHANGE

- Medical schools are now producing 65% more graduates than 5 years ago (up to 6200 per year in 2004), meaning jobs are much more competitive.
- The introduction of Foundation Programmes has made it impossible for consultants from every single speciality to be part of a panel.
- Increasing awareness by Trusts of the importance of checking information provided, to reduce liability and ensure quality.
- Recognition across the medical HR world that other forms of selection, as used in parallel sectors, might be useful and informative in selecting doctors.
- Foundation Trusts have been introduced, which allow the potential for discretionary pay and other terms for doctors.

PREDICTIONS FOR THE FUTURE

Crystal-ball gazing is always dangerous. But picking up trends developing now and looking at my own workload, I make a number of predictions on how the job-seeking process might change. The reasons for these predictions are clustered under discrete objectives.

A need to reduce bias

A test case could question the basis of selection in the medical profession. The process has enormous potential for bias and in every other sector that I have consulted in the rules are much stricter. At the very least, I believe interviewers will be required to take notes, or even record the reasons why individuals were not shortlisted and were not selected at interview. These notes would be available to the candidate.

The wider involvement of non-medical people in the medical profession

The agenda for change has been driven by a justifiable and widespread concern that the medical profession is too secretive and not open enough. 'Lay people' have been introduced at every stage to try to ensure openness. I think it likely that lay people will be required at every interview process. If I were an HR director I'd insist on it.

We want to get the best doctors

As the number of medics in the workforce increases, it is in the interests of Trusts to work harder to get the best available. It isn't just a question of filling a vacancy. Trusts need to perform well and increasingly they understand that hiring and developing the best staff is the surest way to first-class performance. Because the current process is so hit and miss it is likely to be part of a wider review by more ambitious Trusts as they seek excellence.

The realisation that the process does not test how well the doctor can do the job

Neither the CV nor the interview actually tests the ability of an individual to be a doctor. Sales staff have to demonstrate sales technique at selection and managers the ability to manage. Why shouldn't doctors be tested on their ability to be a great doctor? Assessment centres will be used more and more to test a doctor's ability. Mock outpatients clinics and ward rounds would perhaps be too complex to organise. But in-tray exercises and problem solving are not: they could be introduced more widely to good effect.

A recognition that consultants might not be the most appropriate interviewers

It is common practice at the moment for the consultants for whom the doctor is going to work to interview. But there are reasons why this will change:

- Foundation programmes involve too many consultants for them all to be involved.
- Shift patterns mean that Trusts employ SHOs to work across a range of specialities.
- Interviewing is a skilled art that some consultants excel at. Better choices might be made on someone else's behalf by these experienced individuals.
- Other forms of selection don't require a consultant to be present.

The need to remove archaic and unfair parts of the process

Probably the best example is the bullying way in which some consultants insist on a 'Yes' at the end of the interview if they have decided to offer you the job. Unfair, unjust and probably illegal, this will need to stop. If additional stages of the process are introduced (like presentations, written answers, OSCE interviews, selection testing, psychometrics and group and in-tray exercises) then it won't be possible to give an answer at the end of the afternoon.

Summary

- The CV and interview are currently the only forms of assessment used but patterns are emerging which predict significant change over the next few years

- The objective of any such changes shouldn't be to make the process overcumbersome but to make a better decision, and to allow both sides to feel happy with that decision

Medical grades

This is a summary of the medical grade structure currently operating in the UK and includes the introduction of Foundation programmes.

At present, the training positions are:

Grade	Length (years)	Outcome
Medical school	5 or 6	Provisional GMC registration
Pre-registration house officer	1	Full GMC registration
Senior house officer	2 minimum	College certification (MRCP, etc.)
Various ways to proceed to SpR level including:		
Senior house officer posts	6 months each	
Clinical fellowships*	Usually 1 year	
Locum for service*	6 months+	
Locum for training	6 months+	
Research posts	Vary	
Non-standard grades (see below)		
Specialist registrar	4 to 6 months	Certificate of specialist training
Career grade positions. These include:		
● staff grades ● associate specialist ● clinical assistant ● hospital practitioner		

* Often not recognised as part of certified training.

FOUNDATION PROGRAMME GRADE

These replace the PRHO year, which becomes F1, and the first year of the SHO grade outlined above, which becomes F2.

Foundation programmes include a clear requirement to provide formal training in non-technical parts of the doctor's role. These include:

- communication skills
- teamworking
- introduction to management
- time management
- career development and advice.

NON-STANDARD GRADE (TRUST) DOCTORS

BMJ Careers carried out an exhaustive survey of these posts in a supplement published in late 2003. A quarter of all non-consultant posts that were offered were 'non-standard'. They offer some benefits, most notably clinical experience beyond that offered during the SHO years. But they are unlikely to be approved for training purposes. Don't forget that postgraduate Deans need to approve *every* post, which is then allocated a specific training number.

The following are examples of non-standard jobs:

- fellows
- Trust doctors
- doctor for service
- hospital specialist
- resident medical officer.

It might not be the wrong thing to do to take such a position. In fact, it might be the ideal way to progress into the standard job that you seek. But check carefully before you apply and seek information from the sponsoring Trust and consultants to determine the outcomes you expect from the job.

Where do you go to find a job?

UK DEANERIES

The Deaneries have access to lists of Trusts, jobs available in both hospital and general practice, and links to the contact names of individuals who can help with specific enquiries. At present they are as below:

Deanery	Web site address
Eastern	www.easterndeanery.org
Kent, Surrey and Sussex	www.kssdeanery.ac.uk
Leicester, Northampton and Rutland	www.lnrdeanery.nhs.uk
London	www.londondeanery.ac.uk
Mersey	www.merseydeanery.ac.uk
Northern	www.ncl.ac.uk
Northern Ireland	www.nident.org.uk
North Western	www.pgmd.man.ac.uk
Oxford	www.oxford-pgmde.co.uk
Scotland	www.nes.scot.nhs.uk
South Western	www.swndeanery.co.uk
South Yorkshire and South Humber	www.sypgme.nhs.uk
Trent	www.nottingham.ac.uk/mid-trent-deanery
Wales	ww.uwcm.ac.uk/study/postgraduate
Wessex	www.wessex.org.uk
West Midlands	www.wmdeanery.org

A portal is currently in development to list in one place all jobs available within the NHS for doctors.

As well as the list of Deaneries, *BMJ Careers* provides the most comprehensive listing on a weekly basis. This is available online at: www.bmjcareers.com

Although locum agencies generally provide only temporary posts, which are not recognised as part of training, some have contracts to provide substantive positions also. Check with Medacs, the biggest one, at: www.medacs.com

This isn't intended to be a complete bibliography: the management sections of bookshops have a great number of books on the subject of CV writing, interviewing and how to work through career plans. But here are a few books that I find thought-provoking and add something to the content of this book. None is specific to medicine: the most useful source of more information on CV and interview technique in medicine would be to search the archive of *BMJ Careers*.

The *BMJ Careers* fair is an invaluable source of hints and tips. It is held in London at the end of November each year.

SELECTED BIBLIOGRAPHY

CV preparation

The Ultimate CV Book
Martin Yate
Kogan Page
ISBN 0-7494-3875-4
251 pages

The Perfect CV
Max Eggert
Random House
ISBN 0-09-940619-5
146 pages

Killer CVs and Hidden Approaches
Graham Perkins
Prentice Hall
ISBN 0-273-65246-X
322 pages

Interview technique

Successful Interviews Every Time
Rob Yeung
HowTo Books
ISBN 1-85703-978-5
172 pages

Brilliant Answers to Tough Interview Questions
Susan Hogdson
Prentice Hall
ISBN 0-273-65669-4
182 pages

Job Interviews: Top Answers to Tough Questions
John Lees & Matthew DeLuca
McGraw Hill
ISBN 0-07-710704-7
244 pages

Psychometrics and other assessment tools

How to Master Psychometric Tests
Mark Parkinson
Kogan Page
ISBN 0-7494-3420-1
161 pages

Brilliant Selection Test Results
Susan Hodgson
Prentice Hall
ISBN 0-273-66125-5
225 pages

Psychometric Testing
Philip Carter & Ken Russell
John Wiley & Sons
ISBN 0-471-52376-3
234 pages

British Psychological Society:
www.bps.org.uk

Index

30-second window 103
360-degree evaluation 172–173

A

academic background
    application forms 50, 64–66
    CVs 35–37
    interviews 99
academic posts 143–150
    CVs and application forms 144
    interviews 146–150
    presentations 145–146
academic prizes *see* prizes, academic
academic publications 36–37, 145
academic qualifications *see* educational qualifications
acceptance (of post) 154–155
application, e-mail based 46
application by CV 47–48
application forms 1–5, 44–81, 75–81
    academic posts 144
    achievements
        fixed and variable 56, 59
        non-medical 62
    advantages/disadvantages 54–55, 61–62
    advertisements 45–47
    'big hitters' 60, 61, 68
    closing dates 47
    covering letters 78
    CV links 54–57
    design quality 44–53
    downloaded 46–47
    educational qualifications 68
    e-mail based 46
    information packs 98
    language use, positive power verbs 59–60, 67, 69
    multiple 60–61
    personal statements 52, 72
    presentation/format 59–60, 79–80

application forms *cont'd*
 bullet points 59–60
 inclusion of extra pages 63
 introductions 56–57
 principles 59–60
 questions 49–53, 64–74
  academic background 50, 64–66
  audit experience 50, 67
  clinical experience 50, 66–69
  clinical training 67–68
  communication skills 51, 70, 71
  courses attended 64, 65
  driving status 73
  duties 68–69
  illness absence 73–74
  leadership skills/experience 51, 70–71
  learned body membership 66
  management skills 51, 70–71
  personal criteria 51–53, 71–74
  posters 50, 64, 65
  presentations 50, 64, 65
  prizes and distinctions 50, 65–66
  procedures undertaken 68
  research 50, 64, 65
  salaries 52, 73
  teaching experience 51, 69
  teamworking 51, 70
 selection criteria use 62
 sources 45–47
 time saving strategies 58–59
 trends/patterns identification 44–53
assessment tools/tests 169–174, 186
 preparation for 173–174
 types 170–171
audit experience 50, 67
awards *see* prizes, academic

B

bias in medical selection 177
'big hitters' 26
 academic 31–32, 35, 38
  see also prizes, academic
 CVs 21–23
 use at interview 99, 107–108, 121
 use in application forms 60, 61, 68

BMJ Careers 45, 46, 166, 184, 185
book credits 36
bullet points 13, 28, 59–60

C

career grade positions 181
career progression 1
charitable work 33
chronological gaps (in CVs) 21
clinical experience 50, 66–69, 99
clinical fellowships 180
clinical governance 36, 38–40, 99
clinical training 67–68
communication skills 34, 51, 70, 71, 149
competition, in medical selection 176
consultant posts 48
courses attended 50, 64, 65
covering letters 78
CVs 1–43, 47–48, 75–81
    academic background 35–37
    academic posts 144
    achievements, fixed and variable 26–27, 30–31
    advantages 3
    application forms, links with 54–57
    'big hitters' 21–23
    chronological gaps 21
    covering letters 78
    editing 18, 33
    educational qualifications 26, 30–32, 144–145
    employment history 28–29
    front page 9, 15–24
    GMC registration 24
    interests 33, 41
    language use 18
        positive power verbs 12–13
    length 4, 30, 33
    personal contact details 23–24
    photographs 18
    preparation 185
    presentation/format 8–14, 15–24, 33–43, 79–80
        bullet points 13, 28
        headings 10, 34
        topic order 25–26
        word order 19, 21

CVs *cont'd*
  references 78
  review 77–78
  second page
    clinical governance 38–40
    communication skills 34
    interests 41
    management and leadership skills 34–35
    patient focused skills 34, 40
    presentations 36, 37
    references 41–43
    teamworking 34, 35, 40–41
    transferable skills 34

D

Deaneries, UK 183–184
decision making 99
distinctions 32, 64, 65–66
Doctor 167
driving status 73

E

educational qualifications
  application forms 68
  CVs 26, 30–32, 144–145
e-mail based applications 46
employment history 28–29
360-degree evaluation 172–173

F

fellowships
  clinical 180
  research-linked 143–150
foreign applicants 175–176
Foundation Programmes 26, 176, 178
  medical grade structure 180–181
Foundation Trusts 176

G

GAMSAT (Graduate Australian Medical School Admission Test)
    examination 149–150

general practice posts *see* GP posts
GMC registration 24
GP posts 164–168
   interviews 167
   substantive 166–167
GP registrar year 166
grades, medical 180–182
gradual summation 103

H

handwriting 63
house officer posts 180

I

illness absence 73–74
indemnity information 24
information packs 98
interests 41
internal candidates 99, 101–102, 106
Internet 45–47
interviews 82–163
   30-second window 103
   academic background 99
   academic posts 146–150
   assessment tools 169–174
      types 170–171
   'big hitters' 99, 107–108, 121
   bullying 178–179
   clinical experience 99
   closing and follow up 151–157
   decisions, informing candidates 154–157
   delays 108–110
   documents required 92
   failure at 155–157
   feedback 156
   first impressions 92–93
      personal appearance 94–96
   formats/style 89
      combination 158–160
      OSCE 147–149
      recognition 114–116, 126–127, 136

interviews *cont'd*
  GP posts 167
  gradual summation 103
  internal candidates 99, 101–102, 106
  interruptions during 161
  job success maps 98–99
  myths concerning 85–86
  nerves, control of 83
  panels 89–90
  pitfalls 127–128, 137–138, 160–161
  preparation 87–96
    on the day 91–92, 107–113
    tools 107
  preselection 99–100
  questions 84–85
    aggressive/closed 133–142, 158
    final 151–153
    open/retrospective 114–123, 158
    topical 124–132, 158, 167
  selection
    factors influencing 97–106
    panels 104–106
    theory 102–103
  silences during 160
  stress associated 83, 93–94, 107
  success at 154–155
  teamworking presentation 99
  technique 108, 110–113, 120–122, 186
    improvement strategies 129–131, 133, 140–142, 162–163
  transport to 92
in-tray exercises 173

J

jargon 125, 131
JFK question 72–73, 118
job acceptance 154–155
job success maps 98–99

L

language issues 175–176
lay people, medical selection involvement 177
leadership skills/experience 34–35
  application form questions 51, 70–71
  assessment tools 172–173

learned body membership 66
locum agencies 184

M

management skills 34–35
  application form questions 51, 70–71
  interview presentation 99
Medacs 184
medical grades 180–182
medical selection
  application forms *see* application forms
  bias in 177
  competition in 176
  criteria identification 62
  CVs *see* CVs
  future trends 175–179
  interviews *see* interviews
  lay involvement 177
  panels 104–106
motivation 34
multiple consultants panels 104
multiprofessional panels 104–106
multiprofessional work 40–41
  see also teamworking
Myers–Briggs indicator 171

N

networking 40–41
non-standard grade posts 181–182
numerical reasoning assessment 170, 173–174

O

objective structured clinical examinations (OSCEs) 147–149
'over applying' culture 55–56
overseas applicants 175–176

P

panels, medical selection 104–106
  see also interviews

patient focused skills 34, 40
personal appearance 94–96
personal criteria
    application form questions 51–53, 71–74
    CVs 23–24
personality testing 171–172
personal statements 52, 72
photographs (with CVs) 18
positive power verbs (PPVs) 12–13, 59–60, 67, 69
post acceptance 154–155
posters 50, 64, 65
PPVs (positive power verbs) 12–13, 59–60, 67, 69
prejudice 2
presentations
    academic posts 145–146
    application form questions 50, 64, 65
    CVs 36, 37
    skills 146–147
PRHO posts 65
prioritisation assessment 173
prizes, academic
    application form questions 50, 64, 65–66
    CVs 27, 32, 36, 38, 145
procedures undertaken 68
psychometrics 171–172, 186
publications, academic 36–37, 145

R

references 41–43
registration, GMC 24
research background, application form questions 50, 64, 65
research posts 143–150
RITA (record of in-service training assessments) 3

S

salaries 52, 73
selection *see* medical selection
self-motivation 34
senior house officer (SHO) posts 47–48, 180
    presentations 65
    selection criteria 62
    switching to GP training 165–166

shortlisting 149–150
skills, transferable 29, 34
spatial reasoning assessment 171
specialist registrar (SpR) posts 26, 31, 47–48, 181

T

teaching experience 51, 69
teamworking
  application form questions 51, 70
  CVs 34, 35, 40–41
  interview presentation 99
30-second window 103
360-degree evaluation 172–173
time management skills 34, 173
training 67–68
transferable skills 29, 34

V

verbal reasoning assessment 170, 173
visual aids 147
vocational training schemes (VTS) 164–165, 166

W

written answer stage 149–150